ADULT HEMIPLEGIA: EVALUATION AND TREATMENT

Adult Hemiplegia:
Evaluation and Treatment

BERTA BOBATH,

MBE, FCSP, PhD (Hon Boston)

Co-founder, The Bobath Centre, London

THIRD EDITION

HEINEMANN MEDICAL BOOKS

Heinemann Medical Books
An imprint of Heinemann Professional Publishing Ltd
Halley Court, Jordan Hill, Oxford OX2 8EJ

OXFORD LONDON SINGAPORE
NAIROBI IBADAN KINGSTON

First published 1970

Reprinted seven times

Second edition (reset) 1978

Reprinted twice 1979

Reprinted 1981, 1982, 1983, 1984, 1985, 1987, 1989 (three times)

Third edition (reset) 1990

British Library Cataloguing in Publication Data
Bobath, Berta
   Adult hemiplegia. – 3rd ed.
   1. Man. Hemiplegia. Physiotherapy
   I. Title
   616.8′37062

ISBN 0–433–00098–8

Typeset by R. H. Services, Welwyn, Hertfordshire
Printed and bound in Great Britain by
Redwood Press Limited, Melksham, Wiltshire

CONTENTS

FOREWORD TO THE FIRST EDITION

It is often said that in neurology there is accurate diagnosis, but no treatment. The truth is that neurological treatment mainly consists of physiotherapy, adaptation to enforced changes in posture and movement, and re-education. It seems unlikely that there will ever be a drug that will undo the results of a stroke or the degeneration of masses of nerve cells, and so the treatment of neurological disorders will always be in the hands of physiotherapists.

When the doctor meets a patient with hemiplegia, he first tries to find out the cause. When he has done that, and has treated the condition giving rise to the hemiplegia — this may prevent further damage to the brain — the problems of managing hemiplegia remain. Whether the doctor knows he is doing so or not, he chooses either a policy of persuading the patient to use the hemiplegic limbs and retrain his affected side, or else a policy of encouraging the patient to neglect the hemiplegic side and to use the unaffected side for all tasks previously done by the limbs of both sides. The choice affects only the upper limb and the general posture of the patient. There is no choice about the lower limb; the patient has to learn to use it. That being so, it is best for him to learn to use it properly. If the patient gives in to his neurological disorder, he will become an invalid. If he learns to train his hemiplegic side, he returns to life.

There are some less important factors than the patient's ability to live a rewarding life with hemiplegia; there are the social and cosmetic aspects of his case. The more normal the patient can be and can appear, the more satisfactory will be his adjustment within his family and in his social life. The more normal his walking and his standing, the less likely it is that he will be treated as an invalid and that he will become one.

In her book, Mrs Bobath concentrates on the first of these alternatives, that is, on the retraining of the affected side. The success she has had in training hemiplegics has made it obvious to her, and also to those who have worked with her, that this is the best policy: her book will persuade everyone that it is so.

Her method of examining the patient tells us far more about his disability and about his prognosis than does the routine clinical examination of the motor system.

What are the principles of treatment that she has worked out? The physiotherapist's task is to change the abnormal patterns of posture and movement. It is impossible to superimpose normal patterns on abnormal ones, and so the abnormal patterns must be suppressed. The therapist changes the abnormal patterns at their most important points, at what are called key points of control. A change at these points induces a pattern of total posture which is the opposite of that of hemiplegia. First the patient has to learn to hold his head in the correct posture; from the control of the head and neck, the control of the trunk and limbs follows. With the help of the physiotherapist the patient learns to control the patterns himself. All the movements must be done without effort. Excessive effort is worse than useless in spastic conditions, for it reinforces the abnormal patterns of posture and movement and increases spasticity. This form of physiotherapy treats the patient as a whole; it is not treatment for fingers or for a hemiplegic limb.

I am glad to say that among those who are concerned in the treatment of neurological patients, Mrs Bobath's work is already well known. Those who do not know about the rehabilitation of the hemiplegic patient can learn here about a new and successful way of making the best of hemiplegia; those who know something of Mrs Bobath's methods now have a book to instruct them in the total management and treatment of the patient.

P.W. NATHAN

PREFACE TO THE THIRD EDITION

The first edition of this book was written in 1970 after I had developed and tried out treatment and had noted its effect on my patients for 30 years. At that time I had only just started to teach postgraduate courses. The second edition, in 1978, was an attempt to define and describe the treatment in the way I taught it, so that it would be a help for my course instructors as well as for the practising therapists.

The third edition shows the continuation and further development of the treatment, although the underlying concept on which it is based has not changed. However, the emphasis on treatment is now more on the active participation of the patient with the therapist to learn to control his spasticity himself. It means that the patient develops and increases inhibitory control over abnormal tonus and movement patterns. Tonus and movements of the limbs can be most effectively changed and influenced by movements of the spine with its connections to the shouldergirdle and the pelvis. All patients with hemiplegia can move their head and trunk at will and this ability can be utilized in treatment. However, movements of the limbs against the trunk present great difficulties. We have known, and used for a long time, the fact that movements of the trunk against the limbs are much more effective in reducing spasticity than moving an arm or leg against a stable trunk, especially if spasticity is strong. There is now a still greater emphasis in treatment on the role of active movements of the trunk against the patient's limbs. New ways of activating the patient through movements of the trunk have been found, combined with the inhibition of the spastic patterns of the limbs distally by the therapist. In this way, the therapist controls and inhibits spasticity, while the patient remains active and participates with movements of the trunk. When tonus and movements of the limbs are improving, the patient is encouraged, and made, to control movements more and more distally, while the help of the therapist is gradually reduced.

In patients who can sit unsupported, or who can stand, treatment in supine has been reduced, because the patient may be less alert and cannot see well enough what is happening during treatment. This makes his co-operation more difficult. However, treatment in supine remains part of learning to roll over, and for sitting up and lying down. It is also easier for the patient to learn to lift and hold the arm against

'To my husband'

INTRODUCTION

The Bobath treatment has undergone many changes from the time of its inception, but the underlying concept has not changed. It has been evolved for patients with lesions of the upper motor neurone such as for hemiplegia and for children with cerebral palsy. The main problem of these patients is that of abnormal coordination of movement patterns combined with abnormal postural tonus (Bernstein, 1967). Problems of the strength and activity of individual muscles and muscle groups we see as secondary to that of the coordination of their action. We are dealing with a central nervous system which is functioning abnormally, i.e. with lack of control of muscle function. Muscles are the tools of the nervous system and, therefore, the activity of individual muscles and muscle groups is secondary to that of their coordination in patterns of activity. Thus, the assessment and treatment of the patient's motor patterns is the only way of leading directly to functional use. In the hemiplegic patient, muscles are not paralyzed and deficits of muscular activity can be remedied by their action in more normal functional patterns.

This is still the concept of treatment and, hopefully, will not change. What has changed is that we have found new techniques. We have discarded all static ways of treatment like 'reflex-inhibiting postures', but have introduced a strong emphasis on movement and on functional activity. From the beginning the concept has been, and still is, a holistic approach, dealing with patterns of coordination and not with problems of muscle function. It involves the whole patient, his sensory, perceptual and adaptive behaviour, as well as his motor problems. This holistic concept must not be forgotten with the recent tendency to divide the patient's body into parts, such as upper and lower extremities, or hand and foot function, to make research and teaching easier, thus neglecting the interaction of all parts of the body.

We all learn and change our ways of treatment according to our growing knowledge and experience of the reactions of our patients during treatment, for better or for worse. Such changes are good and necessary and will continue. But the concept from which they have evolved should remain intact and should be built upon and enlarged. Changes should advance treatment and not be retrograde by going back to static ways of treatment with emphasis on 'positioning' and by explaining and treating patient's problems of coordination and control of his movements in terms of deficit of muscle function.

In order to avoid the clumsy construction of he/she, I have chosen to designate the patient as 'he' and the therapist as 'she', but obviously the sexes are often reversed.

1

THE NATURE OF THE HANDICAP OF PATIENTS WITH BRAIN LESIONS SUCH AS ADULT HEMIPLEGIA

NEUROPHYSIOLOGICAL CONSIDERATIONS

The physical handicap resulting from a lesion of the upper motor neurone is seen in terms of an interference of normal postural control. We are dealing with abnormal coordination of motor patterns. If we speak of 'patterns of coordination', we mean the patterns of normal and abnormal postural control against gravity. The patient's fundamental problem is seen in abnormal patterns of coordination in posture and movement and in abnormal qualities of postural tone and reciprocal innervation.

Sherrington (1947) states that normal movements need a background of normal tonus. It has to be of moderate intensity, i.e. not too high as to interfere with movement, but high enough to make movement against gravity possible. Tonus and the coordination of movements are indivisible; they depend on each other. Bernstein (1967) says:

> 'Not a single case of pathological coordination is known in which there is not at the same time a pathology of tonus, and that not a single central nervous apparatus is known related to one of these functions without being related to the other.'

The abnormal types of postural tone and the stereotyped total motor patterns we see in our patients are the result of disinhibition, i.e. of a release of lower patterns of activity from higher inhibitory control. Such release does not only produce muscular signs, such as exaggerated stretch and tendon reflexes, but abnormal patterns of coordination, perhaps philogenetically older postural reflex mechanisms. Magoun and Rhines (1946, 1948) have shown that spasticity is due to a release of a facilitatory centre within the reticular substance of the brain stem acting on the Gamma system from higher inhibitory control. Flaccidity, on the other hand, is due to excessive inhibition of Gamma activity from the cerebellum with lack of postural tone against gravity. In both instances, the patient's movements and control of gravity suffer from interference.

Inhibition is a very important factor in the control of posture and movement. Both phylogenetically and ontogenetically it is responsible for the modifications of the total patterns of movement into the selective movements of higher integration. Coghill (1954) has shown that the embryo responds to a stimulus by a movement involving its whole musculature in total patterns. With increase of inhibitory control of the maturing brain, the organism increasingly gains more selective control of posture against gravity. This process follows a cephalocaudal direction, both phylogenetically and ontogenetically. Although the limbs and parts of the body achieve a partial independence in this way, their emancipation from the total pattern is never complete. The movement of a limb remains to some extent always subordinate to the control of the whole organism. The action of the total pattern has to be inhibited prior to the initiation of a localized action. This means that normal functional and skilled activity are largely a matter of inhibitory control. The development is closely associated with the gradual improvement of postural control against gravity. In fact, the long drawn out process of child development can be summarized as due to the maturation of posture against gravity in association with fractionation of the total patterns. Gatev (1972) when writing about the role of inhibition in the development of motor coordination states: 'Imperfect coordination is due to insufficient development of inhibitory activity.' The quality of coordination and its development in early childhood depends, therefore, on increase of inhibitory control and not on increase of muscle power.

Inhibition is active at every level of the CNS. The difference between lower and higher levels of integration is only a matter of complexity. At the spinal level it manifests itself in large patterns of activity, i.e. in total synergies of flexion or extension, such as the flexor withdrawal reflex and the extensor thrust. At higher levels of integration of the CNS, up to the highest one of conscious control, inhibition becomes more and more complex and allows for the fractionation of the original primitive and more total patterns of movement. Selective movements of parts of the body and limbs need inhibition of those parts of patterns which are unnecessary for a specific function. Such fragmentation makes for the great variety and infinite number of new combinations of parts of patterns to be adapted to functional skills. Inhibition does not only make selective movements possible, but plays an important role in the grading of movements, i.e. it is an important factor in 'reciprocal innervation'. It is the balanced activity of excitation and inhibition during a movement which controls its speed, range and direction. Sherrington (1947) states that inhibition is an active process exerted by the CNS which reacts to stimulation with a mixture of inhibition and excitation. Inhibition acts on excitation and changes and moulds it for the purpose of coordination. It modifies and controls action. One might say that inhibition *is* control. It enables us to stop or control action in spite of excitation. Eccles (1973) says:

'I always think that inhibition is a sculpturing process. The inhibition, as it were, chisels away at the diffuse and rather amorphous mass of excitatory action and gives a more specific form to the neural performance at every stage of synaptic relay. Removal of inhibition causes excitation by a process that is called disinhibition.'

The brain-damaged patient suffers from a lack of inhibitory control over his movements. This shows itself in the release of tonic reflex activity, i.e. spasticity, in abnormal total patterns, as well as in his disability to perform selective movements. The patient, as a result of his brain damage, is more or less dominated by his released abnormal reflex activity which interferes with normal activity. Few patients are, even at rest, totally governed by this released abnormal reflex activity, but it will assert itself with any attempt at activities which are beyond his tolerance of stimulation as the result of lack of inhibitory control. This lack of inhibition affects the patient both physiologically and psychologically. It is more difficult to exercise if the individual is excited. With excitation, tonus increases even in the person with a normal CNS, but a normal person can respond with normal coordination of motor patterns.

However, we all know the effects of excitation on the patient with spasticity due to lack of inhibitory control and its effect on both his physical and psychological state. Spasticity will increase, producing deterioration of his movements. Movements become slowed down, laboured, or he may become too stiff to move altogether. Fear, frustration, problems of communication and even meeting a strange person, play a role in making the patient tense and increases his spasticity. Some examples of how the patient can be taught to develop his own inhibitory control over his spasticity are shown in the figures on pp. 62–65.

Some degree of spasticity is found in almost every patient with hemiplegia, and it creates a major problem in the management of the patient. Severe degrees of spasticity will make movements impossible; moderate spasticity will allow for some slow movements, but they will be performed with too much effort and with abnormal coordination; mild spasticity will allow for gross movements with fairly normal coordination, but fine and selective movements of segments of a limb will be impossible or will be performed clumsily. This indicates the intimate relationship between spasticity and movement, and points to the fact that spasticity must be held responsible for much of a patient's motor deficit.

Flaccidity also presents problems, especially during the first weeks after a stroke. In some cases, it may last only a few days, in others for weeks while, in a few cases, flaccidity may persist indefinitely. It then usually affects only the arm, and signs of spasticity will still be found in the wrist and fingers. Only very rarely does the leg remain flaccid as, for instance, in the very old and confused patient who is permanently bedridden.

The clinical neurologist looks upon spasticity as a local muscular phenomenon, and tests it by assessing the degree of resistance a muscle gives to passive stretch. Here, the characteristics of spasticity are seen to be 'exaggerated stretch response', 'the clasp-knife phenomenon' and 'lengthening and shortening reactions'. This view has been supported by the discovery of the dual innervation of muscle, i.e. the alpha and gamma system. Spasticity is now considered to be due to the release of the gamma system, and very rarely the alpha, from higher inhibitory control. This view of spasticity, as a local muscular phenomenon, provides the basis for treatment which aims at the avoidance of exaggerated stretch responses by the use of splints or braces, and of transplants of tendons and other surgical techniques. (Reduction of spasticity has been obtained by intrathecal injections of solutions of phenol; Kelly and Gautier-Smith, 1959.) Injections of dilute alcohol or phenol into the motor points of spastic muscle also promote relaxation, although without permanent effect (Gautier-Smith, 1976). Reduction of spasticity can also be obtained by drugs.

However, when observing a spastic patient, one is struck by the fact that spasticity shows itself in definite patterns of abnormal coordination and that it is not confined to a few isolated muscles. The patient's posture and movements are stereotyped and typical, and he is more or less fixed in a few abnormal patterns of spasticity which he cannot change or can do so only with excessive effort. Therefore, movements, which need a constantly changing background of postural control and adjustment, are prevented. To think of posture as separate from movement is highly artificial, for posture is, in fact, in constant flux and should be regarded as 'temporarily arrested movement' (Bobath, K. 1980).

Reciprocal Innervation

The importance of reciprocal innervation for normal motor activity has been stressed by Sherrington (1913). He studied the interplay of opposing muscle groups on spinal animals in the flexor withdrawal reflex. He showed that an adequate stimulus produced excitation of the flexor groups of muscles of an extended leg with simultaneous inhibition of the antagonistic muscle groups. He stated that inhibition was an active and central phenomenon exerted by the central nervous system and called it 'reciprocal inhibition'. He also stated that reciprocal inhibition in a spinal animal was an artefact not likely to occur in normal circumstances. In the intact organism, spinal inhibition becomes modified by higher central nervous influences and allows for 'reciprocal innervation', a more adequate response to the multitude of stimuli which enters the central nervous system in normal conditions of life. Agonists, antagonists and synergists are pitted against each other in a finely graded way giving the necessary interplay of muscle groups for fixation with mobility and optimal mechanical conditions for muscle power. In normal circumstances all the required degrees of reciprocal interaction in various parts of the body and limbs necessary for postural fixation, grading of movement and for the maintenance of equilibrium are present.

In some traumatic cases of hemiplegia, involvement of the cerebellar system results in motor ataxia which adds to the difficulty of coordination for the hemiplegic patient. Here we find a deviation of reciprocal innervation towards complete reciprocal inhibition. The patient's movements become uncontrolled, excessive in range, and without control of intermediate positions. Volitional attempts to cope with this problem then result in intention tremor or dysmetria.

The aspects of disturbed reciprocal innervation described above are responsible for the way in which a patient is fixed in a few abnormal patterns, and for the difficulty in coordinating movements and their grading. The degrees of fixation in stereotyped postural patterns depend on the severity of spasticity in the individual case and are the result of the release of abnormal postural reflexes which interact with each other.

Treatment aims at the inhibition of abnormally released patterns of coordination and the facilitation of the higher integrated automatic reactions of normal postural control and of those of more voluntary activity. Treatment helps the patient to develop and increase his control over the disinhibited action of tonic reflex activity by use of patterns which inhibit spasticity. Through inhibition his movements are channelled into more normal patterns of function. With the help of the therapist, the patient gains control over the released abnormal non-functional motor patterns.

2

NORMAL AUTOMATIC POSTURAL REACTIONS

Normal postural reflex activity forms the necessary background for normal movements and for functional skills. The basic patterns of coordination which underly and make possible voluntary and skilled activities are those of normal postural reactions against gravity. This normal postural reflex mechanism consists of a great number of dynamic postural reactions which work together, reinforce each other and interact for the purpose of protection against falling and against injury to muscles and joints. They are active during and before a movement is performed, and they give us the ability to counteract gravity without fatigue, and to adjust our posture when we are in an uncomfortable position. They make us able to move in spite of having to keep up against gravity, for instance when walking up and down stairs, or when getting up from a chair or from the floor. They make us change our posture automatically *before* we move in order to make the intended movement possible and easy. We call such postural adjustments 'postural sets'. They are postural changes in anticipation of, as well as accompanying any movement. Horak (1987) says:

> 'Postural adjustments occur not only as a result of sensory feedback in response to unexpected perturbation, but also as a result of "feed forward" in anticipation of expected, self-generated pertubations.'

Postural reactions are active movements, although they are subcortically controlled and automatic. They give us head and trunk control and maintain or restore the normal alignment of head to body and of body to limbs. They also give us the ability to maintain and, more importantly, to regain our balance. Whether they consist of tonus changes only, or can be seen as movements, they are coordinated in patterns which are as complex as those of voluntary movements. There is no dividing line between posture and movement, but only fluid transition from one to the other. Posture is part of every movement, and if a movement is arrested at any stage, it becomes a posture.

The development of coordination in early childhood goes step by step with the development of postural reactions with their appearance, modification and disappearance when more complex and more voluntary skilled activities are acquired. They coincide in time with the various milestones in the child's motor development towards walking and the use of hands for self-help and skills.

The development of automatic control of movement has been called *principal motility* by Schaltenbrand (1927). A knowledge of the development of coordination is necessary for the treatment of all patients with upper motor neurone lesions.

For the purpose of assessment and treatment, three large groups of automatic postural reactions can be differentiated as follows:

RIGHTING REACTIONS

The righting reactions are automatic reactions which serve to maintain and restore the normal position of the head in space (face vertical, mouth horizontal) and its normal relationship with the trunk, together with the normal alignment of trunk and limbs. They develop in childhood and are well advanced at 5 months of age. The movement patterns of these righting reactions are those of our earliest activities, such as turning over from supine to prone-lying and back to supine; raising the head from supine and prone-lying; getting on hands and knees; sitting; and standing up. Rotation around the body axis plays an important role in these activities. These reactions develop in the growing infant, are gradually modified and become integrated into more complex activities, such as the equilibrium reactions and voluntary movement, and are essential in the building up of motor patterns for adult life. Throughout life they are necessary for getting up from the floor, for getting out of bed, for sitting up, for kneeling down, etc.

EQUILIBRIUM REACTIONS

Equilibrium reactions are automatic reactions which serve to maintain and restore balance during all our activities, especially when we are in danger of falling. Their development gradually overlaps with those of the righting reactions. Changes at the centre of gravity necessitate continuous postural adjustments during any movement and even the smallest change has to be countered by changes of tonus throughout the body musculature. The postural adjustments may at times result only in tonus changes invisible to the eye, but they can be noted by palpation or electromyography. If there is considerable displacement of the centre of gravity as, for instance, when there is a danger of falling, the equilibrium reactions are counter-movements of varying ranges to restore the threatened balance. All equilibrium reactions, tonus changes and movements have to be well coordinated, quick, adequate in range and well-timed (Rademaker, 1935; Weisz, 1938; Zador, 1938).

Equilibrium reactions can be tested either by moving the body against a fixed support such as the ground, or by means of a moveable platform or tilting table. We need these reactions when riding on any form of transport. In time, they become so efficient that under ordinary circumstances we are able to maintain our balance with the help of the trunk and lower limbs only, keeping the arms well emancipated and free for skilled manipulative function. Equilibrium reactions involve the patterns of the righting reactions, such as head control and rotation of the trunk and pelvis. They form our first line of defence against injury.

Another important automatic reaction which is closely associated with the development of equilibrium reaction is the 'protective extension of the arms', also called 'parachute reaction'. This reaction serves man's second line of defence in circumstances when equilibrium reactions prove to be insufficient, and the arms and hands are used to protect the head and face from injury when on the point of falling. In the hemiplegic patient, spasticity prevents both groups of automatic reactions from functioning on the affected side. The patient is, therefore, reluctant to carry his weight on that side in sitting, standing and walking.

AUTOMATIC ADAPTATION OF MUSCLES TO CHANGES OF POSTURE

These automatic reactions can be observed in trunk and limbs, and they overlap to some extent with the equilibrium reactions. In a normal person, the central postural control mechanism* governs the weight of a limb during movements both into and against gravity. This mechanism may be called 'postural adaptation to gravity'. Beevor (1904) made the following relevant observations:

> 'In every slow unresisted movement which is made into the direction of gravity, the muscles which act in the direction of the movement are relaxed, whilst their antagonists contract and support the part, and if the movement is continued the latter gradually relax to their full extent.'

He gives the following examples:

> 'The contraction of the erectores spinae, when the body falls forward, occurs automatically and apparently without effort of the will, and it can be demonstrated by leaning forwards, supporting the weight of the body on one hand. On suddenly taking the supporting hand away, the body falls forward and the erectores spinae instantly contract. The contraction is an instinctive preservation action performed automatically, and it always takes place unless a voluntary effort is made to inhibit the contraction when it can be prevented from taking place. In lateral flexion to one side where an obstacle has to be overcome, the rectus abdominis and erectores spinae of that side can be felt to contract together with the external oblique and latissimus dorsi, and probably the quadratus lumborum; but in inclining the trunk to one side — let us say the right —

---

* This term is synonymous with *postural reflex mechanism* as used in the 2nd edition, but we now feel it is preferable because it covers both reflex and voluntary activity.

in the direction of gravity, where no obstacle has to be overcome, the muscles of that side start the movement, but as soon as the centre of gravity of the trunk is displaced to the right of the middle line, the muscles on the right side are relaxed and the muscles of the opposite side (left) — the antagonists — contract, just in the same manner as the erectores spinae contract in flexing the spine forward.'

These studies by Beevor have been confirmed more recently by the electromyographic observations of Clemessen (1951).

A normal person is active when being moved against gravity. Relaxation, unless full support is given, is a voluntary learned ability. If, for instance, the examiner lifts an arm and lets it suddenly go at any stage of the movement, the arm does not fall, but is held and remains in that position for a moment. In this way, the normal person controls every stage of a movement actively and automatically. We call this manoeuvre 'placing'. We use it for assessment and treatment (Figs. 2.1a, b, c). (It is described in more detail on p. 27 under *Normal Postural Reflex Activity*.)

Normal postural control provides three prerequisites for voluntary functional activity.

1. Normal postural tonus of moderate intensity. The term 'postural tone', rather than 'muscle tone', is used here to emphasize the fact that for the maintenance of posture, the CNS activates muscles immediately in patterns involving large groups of muscles. Postural tone must be high enough to resist gravity, but should be low enough to give way to movement.
2. Normal reciprocal interaction of muscles for:
   a. synergic fixation proximally to allow for selective mobility of more distal segments;
   b. automatic adaptation of muscles for postural changes;
   c. graded control of agonists and antagonists integrated with that of synergists for the timing and direction of movement.
3. The automatic movement patterns of the righting and equilibrium reactions which are the background against which voluntary functional activity takes place.

The effect of a lesion of the upper motor neurone can be described as a disturbance of the normal central postural control mechanism. Interference with normal motor ability is caused by a pathological deviation from the three normal fundamental prerequisites mentioned above. Instead of a normal postural tone, we find spasticity; instead of the normal coordination of righting, equilibrium and other protective reactions such as protective extension of the arm against falling (parachute), we find a few static and stereotyped postural patterns. We are dealing with the release of abnormal postural reflex patterns — probably phylogenetically older ones — which give the patient exaggerated static postural patterns with a loss, or inhibition, of the higher integrated statokinetic reactions of righting and equilibrium.

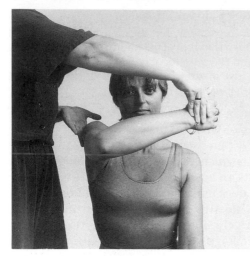

Fig. 2.1a Automatic adaptation
of muscles to changes of posture
(description in text).

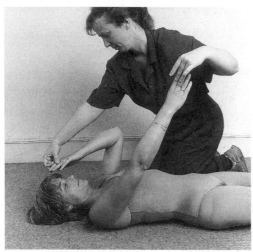

Fig. 2.1b A normal person
controls and—

Fig. 2.1c Follows actively when
being moved.

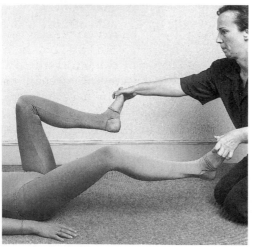

3

ABNORMAL POSTURAL REFLEX ACTIVITY

In the hemiplegic patient the main factors of abnormal postural reflex activity interfering with movement are:

1. Associated reactions;
2. The effect of released asymmetrical tonic neck reflex activity;
3. The effect of released positive supporting reaction.

ASSOCIATED REACTIONS

Associated reactions have been described by Walshe (1923) as tonic reflexes, i.e. tonic postural reactions in muscles deprived of voluntary control. In the hemiplegic patient, associated reactions produce a widespread increase of spasticity throughout the whole of the affected side. This may manifest itself in an accentuation of the hemiplegic attitude. If spasticity is slight or moderate, an excursion of the limb will occur and give the impression of 'a movement', although it is only a change of tonus and not a movement in the strict physiological sense. In patients with strong spasticty, where we find co-contraction of opposing muscle groups, the associated reaction may not produce an excursion of the limb, but can only be detected by palpation. Associated reactions should be differentiated from associated movements (also called synkinetic movements), which are normal and can be seen in young children during their development and also in adults when new and difficult tasks are learned. They are movements of both limbs, the activity of one limb reinforcing that of the opposite side of the body (Fog and Fog, 1963).

Walshe (1923) says:

> 'In none of the flaccid cases examined was any sign of associated reactions in the arm or leg detected. In the spastic cases, a more or less well developed reaction in forceful voluntary activity of the normal limbs was constant . . . The higher degree of spasticity present, the more forceful and the longer lasting will be the associated reactions . . . The response has a comparatively long latent period, is commonly slow in development, and may outlast the duration of the stimulus. The duration of an associated reaction is roughly that of the movement or contraction

evoking it, but there is in some instances a prolonged after-contraction or tonic prolongation of the spasm, which lasts for several seconds. In one case this was still of *undiminished intensity after the elapse of 40 seconds* . . . It may be stated that the more spastic the limb, the longer the latency and after-contraction. It is a fact that antagonistic muscle groups, extensor and flexor, are to be observed in simultaneous contraction.'

Similar ideas have beeen expressed by Nathan (1980):

'Every response is followed by an after-discharge. This affects the muscles which have reacted, and it spreads to involve many other muscles . . . Some of the reasons are the excessive activity of the motoneurones, the increased muscle tone, and the low threshold and excessive and prolonged responses to all stimuli; these features constitute spasticity.'

Associated Reactions and Their Effect on the Patient with Spasticity

Associated reactions are found in all patients with spasticity, not only in hemiplegia, but also in patients with spastic diplegia and quadriplegia. Walshe has described and tested them on the arm of a hemiplegic patient, but they occur throughout all parts of a patient's body which are affected by spasticity. Tonus is changeable with excitation and effort in the patient with spasticity as well as in the normal person. However, in the normal person such increase of tonus is short-lasting and occurs with normal coordination of motor patterns, which are as variable as normal movements. But in the patient with spasticity, increase of tonus due to excitation and effort results in stereotyped abnormal patterns of spasticity, which are long-lasting due to after-contraction. After-contraction is due to lack of inhibition and plays a detrimental role in the performance of repetitive movements. With every attempt at repetition of a movement, the patient's spasticity increases as there is no inhibition between movements. The effect of such after-contraction shows itself clearly in the gradual deterioration of repetitive movements, such as in walking and the use of arm and hand. With the increase of spasticity and co-contraction of opposing muscle groups, the movements are slowed down, smaller in range and performed with increasing effort. The reinforcement and strengthening of the spastic patterns through associated reactions can lead in time to contractures and deformities. Associated reactions may result from any difficulty the patient experiences as, for example, fear of falling due to lack of balance, or becoming agitated when meeting strange people, or, in dysphasic or dysarthric patients, difficulty in communicating. Associated reactions do not only work from the activity of the sound side to the affected one, but also from the affected arm to the affected leg and vice versa. For treatment, this is an indication that the patient should not use any part of his body with excessive effort, and that his balance must be improved to reduce his fear of falling. It is essential at all times to treat the whole patient otherwise, for instance by concentrating on walking without at the same time involving the patient's arm in the treatment, any chances of improving arm and hand function may be lost due to increase of spasticity, or by concentrating on activities of the arm and hand, spasticity of the leg will increase.

In order to reduce the detrimental effect of associated reactions in treatment, the following facts should be considered.

1. There is less spasticity and after-contraction if movements are done slowly, i.e. time is allowed for inhibition between movements.
2. The spread of excitation into total spastic patterns can be counteracted by inhibiting parts of these patterns. In this way, the therapist helps the patient's inhibitory activity and reduces his spasticity.
3. The therapist should inhibit spasticity immediately the movement begins to deteriorate.
4. At the start of treatment, excitation and effort are kept to a minimum, then it is gradually increased, but only as long as the therapist can control the quality of the patient's movement by inhibition.
5. The therapist helps the patient to learn to inhibit this spasticity by the use of selective movements.

THE EFFECT OF RELEASED ASYMMETRICAL TONIC NECK REFLEX ACTIVITY

The asymmetrical tonic neck reflexes, like associated reactions, are released tonic reflexes deprived of higher cortical control. In the spastic patient, they influence the distribution of tonus and the posture of the patient's limbs, the upper limbs more so than the lower. On rotation of the head to one side, extensor tone increases on the 'jaw' limbs and decreases in the 'skull' limbs, with a corresponding increase of flexor tonus in the latter. The strength of the reaction varies with the individual case. In cases of strong spasticity, an immediate response may be seen. On rotating the head to the affected side, the 'jaw' limb extends rigidly, and when the head is turned towards the sound side, the 'jaw' limb flexes. In cases where spasticity is less severe, there may be a delay of a few seconds (latency period of tonic reflexes) and then the reaction sets in slowly and is less strong. Walshe (1923) found the reaction to be more pronounced if the patient turned his head actively, and more so if the rotation was carried out with force against gravity. In many cases, usually those with severe spasticity, the reaction proper cannot be observed and though changes of tone may occur, they are not marked enough to result in a visible movement. The testing of

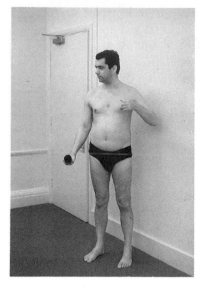 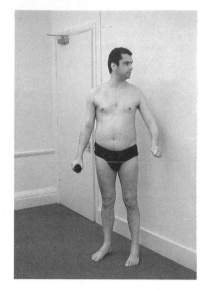

Fig. 3.1a   Patient with moderate degree of spasticity. Interaction of the asymmetrical tonic neck reflex and associated reactions— with head turned to right.

Fig. 3.1b   Same patient as Fig. 3.1a—with head turned to left.

resistance to passive flexion or extension of the limb will, however, reveal these changes of tone. If the arm had flexor spasticity before, it will show decreased resistance to extension on becoming a 'jaw' arm by rotation of the head. The 'skull' arm will show increased resistance to passive extension.

The two tonic reflexes, associated reactions and tonic neck reflexes interact. Thus, when the head is turned away from the involved side and the patient is made to squeeze an object with his sound hand, the flexor spasticity of the arm will become stronger (Fig. 3.1a). But it may extend if the patient's head is turned towards the hemiplegic side while he squeezes an object with the sound hand (Fig. 3.1b).

THE EFFECT OF RELEASED POSITIVE SUPPORTING REACTION

The positive supporting reaction is the static modification of the spinal extensor thrust described by Sherrington (1947) as a brief extensor reaction, evoked by a stimulus of sudden pressure to the pads of the foot and affecting all the extensor muscles of the limb with relaxation of their antagonists.

The adequate stimulus for the positive supporting reaction is twofold:

1. A proprioceptive stimulus by stretch of the intrinsic muscles of the foot, and
2. An exteroceptive stimulus evoked by the contact of the pads of the foot with the ground.

The positive supporting reaction is characterized by the simultaneous contraction of flexors and extensors. The functional grouping of the antagonistic muscles in this reaction differs totally from that taking place in ordinary movements. The antagonists do not relax, but contract, exerting a synergic function, which results in the fixation of the joints (co-contraction).

The normal supporting reaction allows for moderate degrees of co-contraction with the necessary mobility for balance, for movement of the body forward over the standing foot, for mobility of the hip and knee to lift the leg for the next step, and for walking up and down stairs. In the spastic patient, the positive supporting reaction is released from higher control and, combined with extensor spasticity of the leg, becomes an exaggerated spastic response.

SENSORY AND PERCEPTUAL DISTURBANCES

Associated sensory and perceptual disturbances, if present, add considerably to a patient's difficulties. They are a serious handicap to effective treatment and adversely influence the chances of recovery from the functional disability.

In normal movements, there is a close and intimate relationship between the motor and sensory centres of the central nervous system. The influence of sensory and perceptual disturbance on the ability to initiate and perform normal movements is profound. Margaret Reinhold (1951) has stressed that:

'voluntary movement is partly dependent upon

1. the perception of superficial and deep sensation and,
2. motor power and coordination.'

All our movements are performed in response to sensory stimuli which act upon the central nervous system from the outside world through the exteroceptors, especially the distance receptors, eyes and ears. These sensory messsages are integrated at various levels of the CNS and a coordinated response is produced in keeping with the demands of the environment. Movements initiated in this way are then guided throughout their course by a constant feedback (reafference) from the proprioceptors, muscles and joints. From studies of the response of the brain to electrical stimulation, we have become accustomed to thinking of the cortex in terms of localized areas of specific sensory and motor function. However, in the normally functioning organism the cerebral cortex acts as a whole and we should, therefore, think of the sensori-motor areas as one functional unit. This view was expressed by Walshe (1948) when he wrote:

> 'It would seem, therefore, that we may look upon the pyramidal system as an internuncial, a common pathway, by which the sensory system initiates and continuously directs, in willed movements, the activities of the nervous motor mechanism. This sensory affix is a condition of willed movement, and unless we consider both in association, we cannot hope to see the purpose of either.'

Twitchell (1954), also stressed the importance of the integrity of the sensory system for movement and showed that the motor deficit of a limb resulting from complete deafferentation was far more serious than that resulting from ablation of the Rolandic area.

The most frequent sensory and perceptual disturbances are those connected with vision, hearing, proprioception and touch. A common complication of hemiplegia affecting vision is a homonymous hemianopia which may be temporary or persistent. It may be associated with hemianaesthesia or unawareness of the whole of the hemiplegic side. Objects on the affected side may not be seen, or may simply be ignored. The patient will, in general, show little concern either for his inability to move or for the clumsiness of the whole of his affected side. A hemianaesthesia may vary in individual cases from a total loss of perception of the whole of the affected side — even the denial of its existence — to a distortion of the body image affecting only parts of the affected side.

Auditory impairment most frequently takes the form of a lack of comprehension when the patient is addressed. Typically, this may be patchy and fluctuating, varying greatly with the general state of the patient's alertness.

While a right-sided hemiplegia in a right-handed person most commonly produces marked degrees of spasticity and coinvolvement of speech, a left-sided hemiplegia is more often characterized by mild degrees of spasticity, even flaccidity, and with considerable sensory and perceptual impairment.

The impairment of proprioception and touch and other sensations has been described by Brain (1956) as follows:

> 'The appreciation of posture and passive movement is frequently seriously impaired, together with appreciation of light touch and its accurate localization and the discrimination of the duality of two compass points. The appreciation of size, shape, form, roughness and texture often suffers. The qualitative element in pain, heat and cold is still recognized but, in dealing with thermal stimuli in the middle of the scale, the patient may find it difficult to say which of the two is hotter.'

Thalamic or perithalamic lesions usually involve a lack of appreciation of the position of the limbs in space and their relation to the rest of the body. This may affect either the appreciation of a limb position, or the movement of the limb into any one position, or both.

The appreciation of the movement of a limb is less frequently affected than the position in which the limb rests from any length of time.

Cortical lesions produce changes which are often insidious and fluctuating. They vary with the patient's general state of awareness. They reveal symptoms of cortical inattention and extinction — for instance, when identical parts of the arms or legs are touched simultaneously, the touch is appreciated only on the unaffected side, although when tested on the affected side only, touch may be perceived. In the elderly, the handicap is often aggravated by general signs of senility, arteriosclerosis and intermittent periods of confusion. In the early acute phase, these associated sensory handicaps may improve during the first few weeks or months with or without treatment, but for patients with residual hemiplegia, they have a grave influence on both the prognosis of the condition and the effect of treatment.

IMPLICATIONS WITH REGARD TO TREATMENT

The principles and techniques of treatment described later in this book are based on the view that spasticity is caused by the release of an abnormal postural reflex mechanism which results in exaggerated static function at the expense of dynamic postural control. Developed empirically at first, the attempt to describe how the treatment 'works' should be regarded only as a working hypothesis to explain the observed facts (Bobath K., 1980).

The aim of this treatment is to help the patient to gain control over the released patterns of spasticity by their inhibition. This inhibition is obtained by special techniques of handling the patient so as to 'facilitate' the movement patterns of the higher integrated righting and equilibrium reactions, i.e. the static-kinetic movement patterns of the normal central postural control mechanism, which are the automatic background for normal functional skills. Working with various modalities of sensory input, i.e. with specific sensory stimulation such as icing, brushing, vibration or relaxation, etc., as the exponents of certain other treatments recommend, is not, in our view, the answer to the problem. In some hemiplegic patients, even the most searching clinical examination may not reveal any sensory or perceptory impairment. The patient sees and hears, he localizes touch and he can perceive movements and postural changes. But notwithstanding this normal sensory input, the patient can react only with abnormal postures and movements. The reason for this is that the lesion, in effect, 'cuts off' higher integrated activity and produces abnormal motor output, a kind of 'short circuit' into the released abnormal patterns of spasticity. An attempt should, therefore, be made to change the motor output by giving him more *normal sensations* of tonus and movement, and to teach him how to control them unaided. To do this, the patient must be helped gradually to gain control over his abnormal postural reflex activity, to bypass the 'short-circuit' into abnormal patterns, and so to enable more normal motor patterns to become established again.

Experience has shown that there is in every patient some untapped potential for more highly organized activity. The twofold question is how to reach this potential and, if reached, what rational explanation can be given for it.

THE SHUNTING RULE AND ITS APPLICATION TO TREATMENT

The shunting rule of Magnus (1924, 1926) explains, to some extent, how the treatment described in Chapters 5 and 6 works. Its significance for treatment has been stressed by K. Bobath (1959). It was Sherrington, experimenting with a spinal frog, who found that the same stimulus applied within the same receptive field of a particular reflex could produce directly opposite results. For instance, the pinching of the toes of the extended leg of the spinal frog produced a total flexion movement of the leg with flexion and abduction. The flexors of the leg contracted, whereas the antagonists, the extensors, relaxed by central reciprocal inhibition. However, if the leg was originally flexed, pinching of the toes, i.e. giving the same stimulus within the same receptive field produced the opposite result, namely, extension with adduction of the leg. He called this phenomenon 'reflex reversal'. Magnus, on being informed of this observation by Sherrington, made similar observations of 'reflex reversal'. For instance, he examined a cat lying on its side on the table with its tail hanging down over the edge. On pinching the heel of one leg, the tail moved upwards. After placing the cat on its other side, again with the tail hanging down, pinching of the same heel resulted once more in an upward movement of the tail. In looking for a possible explanation for this opposite response, he found the answer in the rule of von Uexküell (1905), who had studied similar responses in lower and primitive organisms such as the Brittlestar or starfish. Von Uexküell stated that in primitive reflex responses the result of stimulation could be predicted with some accuracy. The stimulus favoured the elongated muscle groups, while the contracted and actively shortened muscle groups were in a state of central inhibition.

Based on these experiments, Magnus formulated his 'shunting' rule which went further and can be applied to the motor responses of more highly developed organisms. He stated that at any moment during a movement, *the central nervous system mirrors the state of elongation and contraction of the musculature.* Expressed in a different way, it means that the state of the muscles, therefore, determines the distribution of excitory and inhibitory processes within the central nervous system and the subsequent outflow of excitation and inhibition to the periphery. *It is, therefore, the body musculature which controls the opening and closing of synaptic connections within the central nervous system and determines the subsequent outflow.* Magnus also found that *the greatest effect of shunting is obtained from the proximal parts of the body,* i.e. from the spine, shoulder and pelvic girdles.

In accepting the role of shunting, it is clear that we have a means of influencing and changing motor output from the periphery, i.e. from the proprioceptive system, beginning usually with the proximal parts of the body. By changing the relative positions of parts of the body and limbs when handling a hemiplegic patient, we can change his abnormal postural patterns and stop (inhibit) the outflow of excitation into established 'shunts' of the spastic patterns. We can at the same time direct the patient's active responses into the channels of higher integrated and complex patterns of more normal coordination. In this way, spasticity becomes reduced by inhibition of its patterns, while more normal postural reactions and movements are facilitated.

The ways in which the existing patterns are broken up and resynthesized in different combinations for functional use are described in detail in the chapter on *Techniques of Treatment* pp. 138–139, 'Stage of Relative Recovery'.

4

EVALUATION OF MOTOR PATTERNS FOR INITIAL ASSESSMENT, PLANNING OF TREATMENT AND PROGRESS

There are several concepts underlying the assessment of adult hemiplegia in use today. Their exponents see and interpret the needs of the same patient differently. There is, for example, the 'rehabilitation' concept, with its assessment of functional abilities, or the concept which underlies the assessment of 'ranges of movement' of individual joints, and one which underlies the assessment of 'muscle power'. This book, however, is chiefly concerned with an assessment of the 'quality of motor patterns' and its influence on selective functional activities.

Assessment and treatment should be closely related. A thorough assessment of the problems of each individual patient is a basic necessity if the best results are to be obtained from treatment, and the two should not be regarded as unrelated entities. Treatment should be planned and continued on the basis of frequent and careful assessment. The way in which the problems of the patient are seen, assessed and interpreted should determine the therapist's approach to treatment, her aims in treatment and the choice of techniques used. Many assessment schemes in use today, however, are not related to the methods and aims of treatment, and a valuable aid in planning treatment and giving adequate information regarding treatment results is therefore lost.

Before considering in greater detail the assessment of the quality of motor patterns, it might be of interest to look briefly at the other concepts mentioned above.

The 'Rehabilitation' Concept and Assessment

The 'rehabilitation' concept is concerned with the assessment of the patient's functional abilities, i.e. self-help and daily living activities. Important as this is, it is limited in that it is a quantitative rather than a qualitative assessment. It does not give information about the quality of improvement of function on the affected side, but only a general indication of what activities a patient can do as a whole, with or without the use of his affected limbs. Further, the assessment of functional activities does not in itself give any indication of *how* they are performed; of how much of any activity is done with the affected side; of whether trick or abnormal movements are used, or of the extent to which the sound side is compensating for the affected side. This type of assessment is designed to assess ability, however abnormal it may be, rather than quality of function. It cannot, therefore, give adequate guidance in preparing a treatment plan which aims at improving the functional patterns of the affected side, or in evaluating the quality of improvement achieved.

The Concept and Assessment of 'Joint Range' of Individual Joints

The assessment of joint range of individual joints is based on the concept that passive movements of any joint throughout its range will give reliable information on the patient's ability to use actively the ranges performed passively, should his muscles be strong enough to perform the movement.

This type of assessment is usually done in conjunction with the functional assessment, but is unrelated to it. It does not take into account the effect of *spasticity* on joint range. Where there is no spasticity, joint range in hemiplegic patients is unimpaired, except in a few cases of elderly patients with longstanding residual hemiplegia in whom changes in the joints have taken place. The degree and distribution of spasticity is an inconstant factor. Joint range and limitation of joint range in patients with spasticity are also inconstant and variable. Kelly and Gautier Smith (1959) write:

> 'So far, no objective means of measuring spasticity have been found and clinical observation remains the best method. Range of movement measurements are inaccurate and electromyograph records show much daily variation. The degree of spasticity frequently alters from day to day.'

Furthermore, the assessment of the range of individual joints gives no indication of functional use, as joints which may be fully mobile when moved passively in isolation may present limitations of range when tested in patterns, i.e. simultaneously with other joints. For example, wrist extension may be possible throughout its full range if the patient's fingers and elbow are not extended at the same time, but limited if tested in a pattern of total extension involving the fingers and the elbow. Again, supination may be possible throughout its full range when the patient's arm is in horizontal abduction, but not when it is flexed forward at the shoulder. Or dorsiflexion of the ankle may be possible throughout its full range when the leg is in flexion, but not when it is in extension. In patients with moderate spasticity, dorsiflexion of the ankle may even be obtained with the leg in extension if it is in external rotation and abduction, although not when the leg is internally rotated and abducted.

The Concept and Assessment of 'Muscle Power'

The testing of muscle power of individual muscle groups is based on the concept that either weakness or paralysis of individual muscles is the determining factor in the patient's inability to perform certain movements, or his difficulty in doing so. It leads to the treatment of strengthening the weak muscle groups without finding out the cause of their weakness, or whether it is more apparent than real.

The testing of muscle power of individual muscles, such as is done in poliomyelitis and other conditions of muscle weakness, is unreliable for hemiplegic patients for the following reasons.

1. Weakness of muscles may not be real, but relative to the opposition by spastic antagonists. If the latter's spasticity is reduced, the 'weak' muscles may show normal power. Kelly and Gautier-Smith (1959) discussing the results of intrathecal phenol injections in the treatment of reflex spasm and spasticity, state:

   > 'Many patients are incapacitated by the increase in tone rather than by weakness, and in some, a surprising amount of voluntary power has been unmasked by its reduction.'

   Reciprocal innervation in spastic conditions is not the same as in patients with a normal central nervous system. Contraction of a muscle or muscle group does not result in the normal adapted reciprocal relaxation, i.e. adequate inhibition of their antagonists. Instead, there is exaggerated co-contraction of the opposing muscle groups. This is reinforced by the tonic stretch reflex that makes the elongated antagonists respond with abnormally strong and sustained contraction. This explains the apparent weakness of the prime-movers. Co-contraction shows itself most clearly proximally. Distally, we usually find reciprocal tonic inhibition where one group of muscles is spastic and inhibit the action of their antagonists completely. In some patients with a low postural tone, there is an element of reciprocal inhibition and a lack of co-contraction which makes adquate control of the movement impossible.

2. A muscle that seems to be too weak to contract sufficiently when tested by itself as a prime mover may be capable of strong contraction when acting in a mass pattern (Gardiner, 1963), for instance as part of abnormal tonic reflexes (Brunnstrom 1956, a, b, 1970; Bobath, 1980).

3. Weakness of muscles may be due to sensory deficit, either tactile or proprioceptive or both. With adequate and strong sensory stimulation, apparently weak muscles can be made to contract effectively.

4. Weakness of muscles in hemiplegia and the need for strengthening exercises is seen by us as a secondary problem. The main

problem is their abnormal coordination for postural control and movement. Although atrophy of muscles through inactivity can develop very quickly in some traumatic and in orthopaedic conditions, especially after long-term immobilization in casts and braces, it is rare in cases of spasticity, where the peripheral nerve supply is intact and the circulation to muscles is not obstructed. Here disuse atrophy usually develops late, if at all. We have seen patients with long-standing hemiplegia, with strong spasticity and co-contraction, who had well developed muscles and yet were unable to use them for movement.

THE CONCEPT WHICH UNDERLIES THE ASSESSMENT OF MOTOR PATTERNS

The assessment of the patient's motor patterns as described below is a qualitative rather than a quantitative assessment. It is based on the observation of the patient's motor function on the affected side (Jensen, 1989).

Abnormal coordination is seen as the main difficulty of the patient with hemiplegia and, therefore, the assessment of this coordination is of the utmost importance. The problems of coordination in the hemiplegic patient are similar to those found in other patients with upper motor neurone lesions and many of the tests given in the latter part of this book can also be applied to these conditions.

As has been mentioned above, limitation of joint ranges and weakness of muscles are seen as secondary problems. They are symptoms of the patient's abnormal coordination in posture and movement, i.e. as abnormal patterning of muscle action. Spasticity shows itself in typical patterns produced by interaction of various released tonic reflexes. On the other hand, flaccidity is the result of the lack of postural reflex activity against gravity; tonus is too low and there are no patterns of activity, neither normal nor abnormal. In many cases, we find a mixture of spasticty and flaccidity, for instance, released tonic reflex activity with spasticity in the leg and a lack of postural tone and of normal postural reactions in the flaccid arm. Normal postural reactions need normal postural tonus. However, normal postural tonus is the result of normal postural reactions and, therefore, in obtaining these normal postural reactions in treatment, spasticity can be decreased and, in flaccid conditions, postural tone increased (Bobath K., 1966; Bobath B., 1969).

The inability of a hemiplegic patient to perform voluntary movements — or his ability to perform them in abnormal ways only — is due to a large extent to the deficit of normal postural reaction patterns. Voluntary movements are not entirely voluntary, but depend and are performed on a background of purely automatic postural control. Critchley (1954) writes:

'. . . all associated muscular activity becomes regulated, though not at a conscious level, so as to form a harmony of movement, of which the prime movers constitute the melody. Thus a synergic unit is achieved. Of this, only the prime movers carry out the deliberate volitional, conscious part of the act, the other components of the movement taking place at varying levels of unawareness.'

The automatic movements of postural adjustment accompany voluntary movements like a shadow. Constantly changing 'postural sets' precede voluntary movements and in this way facilitate their performance.

ASSESSMENT OF POSTURAL TONE AND MOTOR PATTERNS

The doctor's medical examination will give the therapist all necessary information about the patient's clinical status, but this will not be sufficient to help in the making of a treatment plan. For this purpose the therapist will need to make her own initial assessment, not only of what the patient can do, including the way in which he moves, but also of what he cannot do. She should discover how much he compensates with his sound side; whether he really needs as much compensation as he uses; whether he could learn to compensate less or in better ways. In other words, it is advisable and necessary to find, obtain and develop any potential of the involved limbs which is being neglected. If the desired function is abnormal or very difficult to perform — and often it is both — the therapist must find out what interferes with it and makes it difficult or impossible. Usually, it is due to release of tonic reflex activity associated with spasticity and abnormal reciprocal innervation. But there is also the problem of loss of memory of former movement patterns and sensory deficit. These problems are closely related and it is important to realize this when making an assessment and planning treatment. The first initial assessment provides a useful basis against which, at later stages, the patient's condition can be compared. But assessment does not stop there: it is an essential part of each treatment session, for assessment and treatment should go hand in hand and they should never be regarded as separate entities. The patient's performance must be assessed continuously during treatment in order to estimate his potential ability and to plan treatment with that aim in view. Constant assessment should make a systematic treatment plan possible, adjusted to the patient's difficulties and needs.

The assessment of the patient's postural and movement patterns gives information about his functional abilities. It is essential to assess not only the motor patterns which the patient needs for specific functional skills, but also his abnormal ones which interfere with them. This gives the therapist a means of planning treatment which aims at giving the patient the wide range of combinations of patterns which are essential for functional use, and at inhibiting those patterns which interfere with normal or more normal function. Functional use needs selective movement, a great variety of motor patterns and a changeable postural background to support these movements. In cases of spasticity, posture is reduced to static function in one or two typical abnormal postural synergies. Muscles can then act only as part of these synergies and for this reason there cannot be adequate functional use. Bernstein (1967) writes:

> 'One is struck by the fact that not a single case of pathological coordination is known in which there is not at the same time a pathology of tonus and that not a single nervous apparatus is known which is related to one of these functions without being related to the other.'

Therefore, the evaluation of the patient's postural patterns also involves that of his postural tone, i.e. of the strength and distribution of his spasticity. As mentioned before, spasticity cannot be measured accurately because it is changeable, its strength varying with the constantly changing state of central excitation of the patient. Its distribution over the body musculature changes with the position of the patient's head in space and in its relation to his body, as well as with the position of the proximal joints of his limbs. The close association of spasticity with the typical abnormal postural patterns of the hemiplegic patient makes a separate assessment of spasticity unnecessary as postural tone and patterns are assessed simultaneously.

SENSORY DEFICIT AND ITS EFFECT ON MOTOR PERFORMANCE

In all cases of hemiplegia it is important to test sensation in order to find out how much of the patient's motor deficit, i.e. loss of motor patterns or weakness of muscles, may be due to sensory deficit. It is also important to repeat sensory tests from time to time in order to find out whether sensory stimulation given in treatment has produced any changes.

A great variety and degree of sensory deficit can be found in these patients, ranging from slight or partial sensory loss to complete agnosia of the affected limbs. The patient may have loss of postural sense and be unable to appreciate passive movements. He may not be able to recognize objects held in his affected hand, or their size, shape or texture. He may be unable to localize touch, pressure or pain, and though he may be aware of the difference between hot and cold, he may not be able to differentiate between degrees of hot and cold.

As mentioned before, in many patients with hemiplegia the motor disturbances are aggravated by sensory impairment. Patients with sensory deficit lack the urge to move and do not know how to move limbs or segments of limbs which they do not feel properly. It is interesting that many patients have more accurate sensory discrimination in the leg and foot than in the arm and hand. A reason for this may be that the leg is used in standing and walking at a fairly early stage, while the hand may never be brought into use at all. Another factor pointing to the inter-relation of sensory and motor recovery seems to be that more accurate localization of light touch and two-point discrimination can be found in the proximal parts of the limbs than in the distal ones. Although the patient with moderate or slight sensory deficit may acquire some of the most essential movement patterns, the patient with severe and persistent sensory deficit has a poor prognosis for functional recovery.

Sensory Testing

Though testing of sensation is usually done by the neurologist, some sensory tests have a specific significance for treatment and should, therefore, be done by the therapist. Retesting from time to time is desirable. Improvement of sensation often occurs as a result of treatment.

Tests for sense of position and appreciation of movement

Both sense of position and appreciation of movement should be tested because the patient may well be able to appreciate a movement, but may not be able to appreciate the position after having been moved and left in that position for a lengthy period of time. One of my patients was able to appreciate the movements of his arm by me, but did not know where it was in bed after sleeping.

Testing can be done with the patient in supine or sitting and often gives better results in sitting. The therapist moves his affected arm, arresting the movement at various stages. First the affected extended arm is moved at the shoulder, and then movements of the elbow, wrist and fingers are added so that a variety of movement patterns are passively performed. The patient is asked to imitate the movements so that he can compare what he is doing with what the therapist has done with his affected arm. He is then blindfolded and has to rely completely on what he feels. After each movement done with his affected arm, the blindfold is removed and he is asked to look and compare the end position of his sound and affected arm to see whether they are the same. In this way testing and training can be combined. Usually movements at the shoulder are better appreciated than those of elbow, hand and fingers. The same tests should be done with his legs and feet. Often the patient's appreciation of his movement and sense of position of the leg and foot is better than those of the arm.

Tests for localization of pressure and light touch

Pressure with one finger on the patient's limbs is usually better appreciated than light touch, and should be done first, i.e. before touching the limb lightly. He is asked to say 'yes' when he feels the touch, which is given at various points of the limb. If there are speech problems, he may be asked just to nod his head. Localization of touch can be indicated by making the patient put a finger of his sound hand on to the point of touch. If localization is disturbed, he usually refers the point of touch proximally, i.e. if the forearm is touched, to the upper arm; if the hand is touched, to the forearm. Appreciation of touch on the fingers is often absent, especially on the fingertips. Often localization of touch is better on the leg than on the arm.

Tests for stereognosis

A normal person when blindfolded manipulates an object given to him in order to recognize it. This the patient cannot do and, therefore, it may help him if the therapist moves the object around in his hand. If he cannot recognize the object, he may be able to say whether it is hard or soft, long or short, smooth or rough, whether it is round or has edges.

TESTING OF TONUS AND POSTURAL REACTIONS TO BEING MOVED

This way of testing is designed to find out why the patient is unable to perform a particular movement and what prevents it. The reactions of a normal person to being moved are compared with those of a patient with hemiplegia. It must be appreciated that tonus and movement are inseparable and can best be tested simultaneously. A person with a normal central nervous system, i.e. normal coordination and tonus, will follow and support actively any movement done with him, especially when moved against gravity. His muscles will adjust themselves actively and automatically to any change of posture or to any movement. He neither resists the movement — unless he resists voluntarily — nor does he relax unless he is fully supported. This automatic adjustment is protective against injury or loss of balance and falling. The patterns of coordination to being moved are the same as when doing an indentical movement voluntarily or on request. This means that the ability to react normally to being moved is a precondition for normal voluntary movements. It shows the presence of a normal postural reflex mechanism with its normal tonus and coordination.

The patient with abnormal coordination and tonus, however, does not adjust himself normally to changes in posture, i.e. to being moved. In the presence of spasticity, there is excessive resistance to being moved *against* the patterns of spasticity on the one hand, and undue and excessive assistance on the other hand, when moved *into* the patterns of spasticity.

As stated above, tonus and movement interact and, therefore, should not be tested and treated separately. Although we cannot see tonus, we can feel tonus changes. We can see signs of spasticity only by its effect on posture and movement. However, we can see and assess movements and their quality. Therefore, we test tonus and movement patterns simultaneously. *We do this by feeling for changes of tonus, while at the same time, observing the patient's movements.*

The hemiplegic patient has lost his normal automatic postural reactions against gravity. When he leans forward in sitting, his trunk flexors contract instead of his erectores spinae and he tends to fall forward and down. When he is made to lean towards the affected side, the side-flexors of his neck and trunk contract on that side, and as those of the sound side do not contract to hold him up, he tends to fall towards the affected side.

The patient has also lost the normal adaptation of muscles against gravity during movements of his limbs. The spastic contraction of the flexors and depressors of the shouldergirdle and of the extensors of the leg suppresses the normal postural activity of their antagonists. Instead of relaxing during a downward movement into gravity, this spastic contraction even increases towards the end of the movement, that is to say it becomes stronger the further the limb is moved in the direction of gravity. This leads to a complete inhibition of the action of the antagonists, i.e. of the muscle groups which should hold and act against gravity and which should afterwards raise the arm or leg. Therefore, the hemiplegic patient cannot reverse the movement of lowering his arm or leg at any given point, least of all at the end of the movement downward. He is unable to arrest the downward movement of the arm or leg at any stage when it is left unsupported. For this reason, it is most difficult for him to lift his arm when it is hanging down or held flexed by the side of his body, or to lift his leg after having it fully extended. The weakness of the flexors of the leg and of the elevators of the arm is relative and in direct proportion to the inhibition imposed upon them by their spastic antagonists. In order to make the patient lift his arm or leg against gravity, we have first to restore the normal reflex mechanism controlling the weight of the limbs against gravity. We may obtain this control by first elevating the arm, or flexing the leg passively, then waiting until there is no spastic resistance to these positions and, finally, moving the limbs downward stage by stage, making the patient hold the limb at every stage and moving it up again if he is unable to hold it. In the end, if the leg can be nearly extended while it is still held and controlled by the patient, or if the arm is almost by his side, the patient not having let it fall, he will be able to lift the leg or arm with ease. When he has gained control and is able to support the weight of his limbs at any stage of a movement, he is able to reverse it and raise the limbs with the action of the same muscles which have been active during the movement downward into gravity.

In addition to being a method of testing, this is an important part of treatment and is called *placing*. To enable the patient to obtain active control, only minimal support should be given when moving the arm, or when moving a leg. In the more advanced patients, who are able to control and use various combinations of movement patterns as needed for functional skills, the therapist should work for 'placing' in different combinations of positions and movements, i.e. in adduction and abduction, external and internal rotation, with flexed or extended elbow, and in supination and pronation.

The therapist moves the patient's body or limbs using exactly the same movement patterns which the patient is expected to perform later on, but which are currently subject to interference by his patterns of spasticity. As the therapist moves the patient's limbs, she tests his adaptation to the normal patterns of posture and movement imposed upon him. As mentioned above, where postural reflex activity is normal and immediate, active adjustment of the muscles to changes of posture occurs, and the patient will follow actively throughout its course any movement done with him by the therapist, provided that only slight support, or rather guidance, is given to the movement. Normally, a person is not 'relaxed' when being moved, but actively controls the weight of his body or limbs. If left alone at any stage of the movement, his limbs do not fall, but automatically remain for a moment before another more comfortable position is assumed, i.e. he rights himself. While being moved, he gives no resistance to the movement performed and his limbs feel light. If the patient should react in this normal way during any phase, or during the whole sequence of a *guided movement*, it indicates to the therapist that he can perform that part of it, or the whole sequence, unaided and in a normal way. If there is *spasticity*, its effect on such a guided movement is twofold:

1. If the movement is performed against the pattern of spasticity there is *resistance*. The degree of resistance encountered by the therapist indicates not only the degree of spasticity but, more important, the degree to which spasticity interferes with the possibility of the movement being performed by the patient unaided. If the resistance is strong, the patient cannot be expected to perform the movement at all. If it is moderate, or if resistance occurs only at some stages of the movement, the patient is able to perform some part of the movement, or even the whole, but only with excessive effort and in an abnormal way. If resistance is slight, the patient is able to perform the movement in a fairly normal manner, but with greater effort and at a slower rate than is normal. Such abnormal resistance due to spasticity is encountered in the arm, hand and fingers with all movements of extension, external rotation, supination and abduction of fingers and thumb, and also with elevation and horizontal ab-duction of the extended arm and hand and with full adduction of the arm with flexed elbow and extended wrist and fingers, as in touching the opposite shoulder. Resistance is also encountered

in bending the elbow when the arm is elevated and when held horizontally forward at the shoulder. In the leg, resistance is encountered with all movements of flexion of the hip, knee and ankle, and dorsiflexion of the toes, as well as pronation of the ankle.

2.   If the movement is performed *into* the direction of the pattern of spasticity, there is uncontrolled *assistance* to the passive, or to the guided, movement. This assistance manifests itself either in a sudden 'pull' due to flexor spasticity, or in a sudden 'push' due to extensor spasticity. If either the flexor or extensor spasticity is severe, i.e. if the pull into flexion or the push into extension is strong, there will be equally strong resistance to the attempt to reverse the movement passively, and it will be impossible for the patient to do so actively. If spasticity is moderate or slight, this uncontrolled and exaggerated assistance may only occur towards the end of the movement. This indicates that although the patient may not be able to reverse the movement after this has happened, he will have some initial range which he can control and within which he can actively reverse the movement.

If there is *flaccidity*, the patient's limbs feel heavy and abnormally relaxed when being moved, and there is no active adjustment of muscles to changes of posture; no active following and controlling of the movement by the patient; and no ability to arrest a movement and hold a posture against gravity when not supported. This indicates to the therapist the absence of normal postural reflex activity and, therefore, the patient's inability to perform the movement unaided and actively.

When testing for postural reactions in response to being moved, the therapist is testing the patient's postural tone as well as his ability to move. Excessive resistance to the movement performed by the therapist indicates abnormal spastic reactions which interfere with the patient's active movements. Lack of postural tone in flaccid conditions shows itself in excessive weight of the body or limbs when being moved without control by the patient. Both abnormal postural reactions and lack of postural reactions, i.e. spasticity or flaccidity, may occur in the same patient in different parts of his body or during different stages of movement.

The patterns of spasticity produce retraction, fixation and depression of the scapula and humerus in the arm, contraction of the side-flexors of the trunk on the affected side, internal rotation of the arm at the shoulder and flexion with pronation of the elbow and wrist, and the hand in ulnar deviation. In some cases, however, there is external rotation of the arm with supination and flexion of the elbow combined with retraction at the shoulder. The fingers are flexed and adducted except in a few cases when they are extended and adducted, which occurs with extreme flexion of the wrist.

The spastic pattern in the leg produces rotation backwards and the pulling upwards of the pelvis on the affected side. Due to the rotation backwards of the pelvis, the leg usually shows a pattern of *external* rotation. This is despite the fact that extensor spasticity is normally combined with *internal* rotation. A change of this pattern of external rotation can be observed if the pelvis is moved forward on the affected side when internal rotation occurs. Extensor spasticity of the leg shows itself with extension of hip and knee, supination of the foot and plantiflexion of the toes.

Tests I and II (pp. 34–58) are to be used as part of treatment as well as for an initial assessment, as they give detailed information about what should be done in treatment. Although testing in this way may be laborious, it is a vital aspect of assessment and treatment, and essential for finding out as much as possible about the needs of the individual patient.

An example of a short initial assessment chart, giving the patient's functional abilities, disabilities and difficulties, and their underlying causes, is given below. It makes a general plan of treatment possible by indicating the patient's main problems and some of his potentials, but cannot be used for ascertaining progress.

SHORT ASSESSMENT AND TREATMENT PLANNING FOR ADULT HEMIPLEGIA

PATIENT'S NAME: A.L.   AGE: 54

ADDRESS: PROFESSION: Housewife

DIAGNOSIS: Left hemiplegia following subarachnoid haemorrhage.

DATE OF EXAMINATION: 17th March, 1985

DATE OF ONSET: 8th October, 1984 (Craniotomy and clipping of anterior communicating aneurysm, 15th October, 1984).

UNDERLINE AND ANSWER 'YES' OR 'NO' WHERE POSSIBLE

1. *General impression of patient*
   Seemingly younger or older than chronological age.
   Co-operation. Indifference, emotional release, depression, negativism, aggression, euphoria, instability.

---

2. *State of health*
   (How careful has one to be.) Hypertension; heart insufficiency; respiration, giddyness, weakness, etc. (Guidance by doctor).
   Circulatory disturbances arm and leg,—D.V.T., (knee swollen) 'Sudek' of hand, stiff metacarpo-phalangeal joints and oedema. General health good.

3. *What can the patient do?*

Does she use her trunk for balance? Does she use her normal side for every activity?

Walks without stick slowly—very stiff, balance precarious. Can dress and undress with little help, feels insecure without supervision.

Could she function with less compensation?

---

4. *What can she not do?*

Use arm and hand for any activity. Has painful and fixed shoulder, painful hand. Cannot stand on left leg only and lift right foot.

Does she *really* need a tripod? an elbow crutch? a stick? a brace? a sling?

No. Perhaps a stick when walking outdoors for balance but not for weightbearing.

Could she learn to walk with or even without an ordinary walking stick?

Yes.

With or without a brace?

Without brace.

Is there potential on the affected side? Arm? Hand? Leg? Foot?

Yes, arm and leg and foot.

Is she still within the period of spontaneous recovery?

Yes.

How is her balance in:

Sitting:

Good, but no arm support left.

Standing:

Little weight on left leg, no balance on left leg.

Walking:

Steps too quick with right foot because no weight on left leg, unstable left hip.

Can she use her affected arm?

No

Her affected hand?

No.

Has she got associated reactions?

Affecting mainly the fingers.

Can she speak?

Yes.

Does she understand language?

Yes.

Can she read or write?

Yes. (she is left-handed.)

5. *The sensory state*
(This is very important because of the effect of sensory deficit on movement, muscle power and prognosis.)
To test:
Deep sensation (proprioception): of arm and leg. Position sense. Appreciation of movement. (Both to be tested separately.)

Arm:

Disturbed—at shoulder, elbow, wrist, and hand—appreciates movement but not direction.

Leg:

Good.

Tactile sensation: on arm and leg. Discrimination of light touch. Pressure, stereognosis, temperature, dermatographia.

Touch diminished below elbow. Astereognosis of hand.

Leg: Good.

---

6. *Tonus*
Test reactions to being moved on arm and leg. Test in supine and sitting.
Spasticity: gives abnormal resistance or exaggerated assistance.
Flaccidity: uncontrolled full weight of limb.
There may be a mixture of both.

Leg:

Extensor spasticity, heavy leg, strong resistance to dorsiflexion—resistance to full extension of knee. Some adductor resistance.

Arm:

Shoulder-pain, medial rotation. Resistance to full passive elevation. Hand very stiff, resistance to flexion of metacarpal-phalangeal joints, semiflexion of distal joints 'Sudek'.

---

7. *What is the most important and first aim in treatment?*

Mobilizing of neck and shouldergirdle to prevent shoulder-pain and pain of hand. Weightbearing on left leg, prevention of contracture of knee.

---

8. *Which function should the patient be prepared for at this stage?*

Control of shouldergirdle and arm, lifting and placing and holding arm up. Active elbow movements, mainly extension. Standing and balance, walking.

---

9. *What may be your final limitations?*

Use of arm and hand. Profound sensory loss. Dorsiflexion of ankle.

10. *What can you make the patient do with little help?*

Nothing with the arm yet.

Take weight on left leg and extend knee.

Stand up from chair without use of right hand.

Walk better with help than without help.

11. *What will you do in treatment?*

1. Mobilize shouldergirdle, work against retraction of the scapula in side-lying, supine, sitting and standing. Get painless elevation of arm in external rotation when scapula is mobile and shouldergirdle forward. Get extension of elbow and holding against intermittent push, alternating with slight flexion.

2. Maintain and increase range of flexion at metacarpal-phalangeal joints.

3. Standing with weight over left leg and hip forward, small steps with right foot forwards and backwards.

TESTS FOR SPECIFIC MOVEMENTS

Two groups of tests which are designed to give information about the patient's ability or inability to perform specific movements, and progress under treatment, are given in detail under the following headings:

I. Tests for the quality of movement patterns.
II. Tests for balance and other automatic protective reactions.

The tests for quality of movement patterns have been divided into three grades according to their degrees of difficulty. The tests for grade 1 are the easiest and those for grade 3 the most difficult. The grading is intended to enable the therapist to limit, initially, the number of tests in the severely affected patient. Gradually, with the patient's progress under treatment, those of grades 2 and 3 may be added. Tests of balance and other automatic reactions can only be attempted in the moderate or slight cases and have not, therefore, been graded.

I. TESTS FOR THE QUALITY OF MOVEMENT PATTERNS

The patient who can move his limbs actively, that is, the patient with moderate spasticity, can only use total flexor and/or extensor synergies. He lacks selective movements. Flexor muscles may contract in total patterns of flexion of the whole limb against the resistance of extensor spasticity, and extensor muscles act only in total patterns of extension against the resistance of flexor spasticity. These two total patterns give limited functional use and abnormal performance in walking, while the use of the hand for manipulation will be altogether impossible.

A somewhat greater variety of motor patterns, but still lacking the necessary independent and selective action of individual segments of a limb for functional use, is possible in cases of slight spasticity, but movements are slow, laboured and clumsy. Dr Denis Williams, lecturing on spasticity said:

> 'If you want to beckon with your index finger, it is not the contraction of the flexor indicis proprius which is of importance, but the inhibition of the total flexor pattern of the arm that makes it possible.'

This example shows clearly the problem of lack of selective movements in the hemiplegic patient. It is the inhibition or, one might say, the fragmentation of the total flexor pattern of the arm which makes selective movements possible, and not the contraction or lack of contraction of a particular muscle or muscle group. The same problem applies to all other selective movements, whether they be independent movements of the ankle or toes, the knee or elbow or of the wrist or fingers.

Functional movements at any level of integration, from the relatively simple automatic postural reactions of righting and balance to the complex and finest selective movements needed for manipulation, need manifold combinations of parts of the more total and primitive movement patterns which are present at early stages of development of coordination. The great variety and manifold combinations of movement patterns necessary for skilled activities depend on the ability of *any* muscle or muscle group to function as part of a great number of patterns and not only as part of one or two total patterns. The tests have been graded, therefore, in such a way as to start with the more simple progressing towards the most selective movement patterns.

I. TESTS FOR THE QUALITY OF MOVEMENT PATTERNS

Patterns to be tested
Tests for Arm and Shouldergirdle (to be tested separately in supine, sitting and standing, as the result will be different in these positions.)

Grade 1	Supine		Sitting		Standing	
	Yes	No	Yes	No	Yes	No
a. Can he hold extended arm in elevation after having it placed there?						
With internal rotation?						
With external rotation?						

Test for Arms and Shouldergirdle—*contd.*

	Supine		Sitting		Standing	
	Yes	No	Yes	No	Yes	No
b. Can he lower the extended arm from the position of elevation to the horizontal plane and back again to elevation? . . .						
Forward-downwards?						
Sideways-downwards?						
With internal rotation?						
With external rotation?						
c. Can he move the extended abducted arm from the horizontal plane to the side of his body and back again to the horizontal plane?						
With internal rotation?						
With external rotation?						
Grade 2						
a. Can he lift his arm to touch the opposite shoulder?						
With palm of hand?						
With back of hand?						
b. Can he bend his elbow with his arm in elevation to touch the top of his head? . .						
With pronation?						
With supination?						
c. Can he fold his hands behind his head with both elbows in horizontal abduction? . .						
With wrist flexed?						
With wrist extended?						

Test for Arms and Shouldergirdle—*contd.*

	Supine		Sitting		Standing	
	Yes	No	Yes	No	Yes	No
Grade 3						
a. Can he supinate his forearm and wrist? . .						
Without side-flexion of trunk on the affected side?						
With flexed elbow and flexed fingers? . .						
With extended elbow and extended fingers?						
b. Can he pronate his forearm without adduction of arm at shoulder						
c. Can he externally rotate his extended arm? (i) in horizontal abduction?						
(ii) by the side of his body?						
(iii) in elevation						
d. Can he bend and extend his elbow in supination to touch the shoulder of the same side? starting with:						
(i) arm by side of his body?						
(ii) horizontal abduction of the arm? . . .						

Tests for Wrist and Fingers

	Yes?	No?
Grade 1		
a. Can he place his flat hand forward down on table in front?		
Can he do this sideways when sitting on plinth? . . .		
With fingers and thumb adducted?		
With fingers and thumb abducted?		

Test for Wrist and Fingers—*contd.*	Yes?	No?
Grade 2		
a. Can he open his hand to grasp?		
With flexed wrist?		
With extended wrist?		
With pronation?		
With supination?		
With adducted fingers and thumb?		
With abducted fingers and thumb?		
Grade 3		
a. Can he grasp and open his fingers again?		
With flexed elbow?		
With extended elbow?		
With pronation?		
With supination?		
b. Can he move individual fingers?		
Thumb?		
Index finger?		
Little finger?		
2nd and 3rd finger?		
c. Can he oppose fingers and thumb?		
Thumb and index finger?		
Thumb and 2nd finger?		
Thumb and little finger?		

Tests for Pelvis, Leg and Foot Prone Tests	Yes?	No?
Grade 1		
Can he bend his knee without bending his hip?		
With foot in dorsiflexion?		
With foot in plantiflexion?		
Foot inverted?		
Foot everted?		
Grade 2		
Can he lie with both legs externally rotated and extended, feet dorsiflexed and everted, heels touching? .		
Hold position when placed?		
Turn affected leg out again to touch heel of sound leg after it has been internally rotated by therapist? . . .		
Perform internal and external rotation unaided? . . .		
Grade 3		
a. Can he keep heels together and touching while bending both knees to right angle?		
Affected foot inverted?		
Affected foot everted?		
b. Can he hold knee of affected leg flexed at right angle and alternately dorsiflex and plantiflex ankle?		
Foot inverted?		
Foot everted?		
Without moving his knee?		
Tests for Pelvis, Leg and Foot **Supine**		
Grade 1		
a. Can he bend affected leg?		

Test for Pelvis, Leg and Foot—*contd.*

	Yes?	No?
With sound leg flexed, foot off support?		
With sound leg extended?		
Without bending affected arm?		
b. Can he bend hip and knee with foot remaining on the support from the beginning of extension until the foot is near his pelvis?		
Can he extend his leg by degrees, his foot remaining on the support?		
Grade 2		
Can he lift his pelvis without extending his affected leg, both feet on the support?		
Can he keep his pelvis up and lift his sound leg? . . .		
Without dropping pelvis on the affected side?		
Can he keep pelvis up and adduct and abduct knees?		
Grade 3		
a. Can he dorsiflex his ankle?		
Can he dorsiflex his toes?		
With flexed leg, foot on the support?		
With extended leg?		
With foot inverted?		
With foot everted?		
b. Can he bend his knee when he lies near the edge of plinth, his leg over side of plinth? (hip extended) . . .		

Test for Pelvis, Leg and Foot—*contd.*	Yes?	No?
Sitting Tests on Chair		
Grade 1		
a. Can patient adduct and abduct affected leg, foot on ground?		
b. Can he adduct and abduct affected leg, foot lifted off ground?		
Grade 2		
a. Can he lift affected leg and place foot on sound knee? (without use of hand to lift leg.)		
b. Can he draw affected foot back under chair, heel on the floor?		
c. Can he stand up with sound foot in front of affected one? (without use of hand?)		
Standing Tests		
Grade 1		
Can he stand with parallel feet, feet touching?		
Grade 2		
a. Can he stand on affected leg, lifting sound one? . . .		
b. Can he stand on affected leg, sound one lifted, and bend and extend standing leg?		
c. Can he stand in step position, weight forward on affected leg, sound leg behind on his toes?		
d. Can he stand in step position, sound leg forward with weight on it, affected leg behind and bend knee of affected leg without taking toes off ground?		

Test for Pelvis, Leg and Foot—*contd.*

	Yes?	No?
Grade 3		
a. Can he stand in step position, weight forward on sound leg, affected leg behind and lift foot without bending hip of affected leg?		
Foot in inversion?		
Foot in eversion?		
b. Can he stand on affected leg and transfer weight over it to make step with sound leg?		
Forward?		
Backward?		
c. Can he stand on sound leg and make step forwards with affected leg without hitching pelvis up?		
d. Can he stand on sound leg and make step backwards with affected leg without hitching pelvis up?		
e. Can he stand on affected leg and lift his toes?		

II. TESTS FOR BALANCE AND OTHER AUTOMATIC PROTECTIVE REACTIONS

As mentioned before, we test the patient's reactions and their quality of coordination when disturbing his balance by moving him. Automatic postural reactions are part of every voluntary movement, forming, in fact, the background on which voluntary movements are performed. The postural reflex mechanism underlying voluntary movements must be normal before the patient can expect to perform normal or more normal movements and skills. The most important of these postural reactions to be tested in the hemiplegic patient are as follows:

Balance reactions

1. Support and balance reactions on the affected forearm or on the affected extended arm when he lifts his sound arm and turns over from prone lying on his side.
2. Balance reactions of the trunk and legs in sitting without the use of his sound hand, weight on the affected hip.
3. Balance reactions in four-foot kneeling.
4. Balance reactions in kneel-standing.
5. Balance reactions in half-kneeling.

6. Balance reactions in standing, feet parallel.
7. Balance reactions in standing, feet in step position.
8. Balance reactions on affected leg when making steps with sound leg.
9. Balance reactions standing on the affected leg, the sound leg lifted.

Protective extension and support on affected arm

1. In being moved forward towards table or wall (Fig. 4.24. p. 55)
2. On being moved sideways to affected side towards table or wall. (Fig. 4.25. p. 57).
3. To protect face with affected arm and hand against ball or pillow thrown against him. (Fig. 4.27. p. 58).

II. TESTS FOR BALANCE AND OTHER AUTOMATIC PROTECTIVE REACTIONS

(*N.B.* In order to test these reactions, the patient must be able to assume and hold the test position. He should react with specific movements in order to regain his balance or protect himself against falling when being moved or pushed unexpectedly. It should be noted that the photographs on pp. 44–58 show normal balance reactions for which the therapist should strive when working with her patients.)

1. Balance Reactions

	Yes?	No?
Patient in prone lying, supporting himself on his forearms.		
a. His shouldergirdle is pushed toward affected side. Does he remain supported on affected forearm? (Fig. 4.1) ...		
b. His sound arm is lifted forward and up, as when reaching out with one hand. Does he immediately transfer his weight towards the affected arm? (Fig. 4.2)		
c. His sound arm is lifted and moved backwards and he is turned to his side, support on affected arm. Does he remain supported on affected arm? (Fig. 4.3) ..		

These three tests can be done in slight cases with patient supporting himself on his extended arm instead of his forearm.

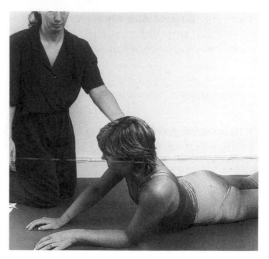

Fig. 4.1

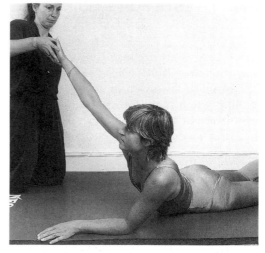

Fig. 4.2

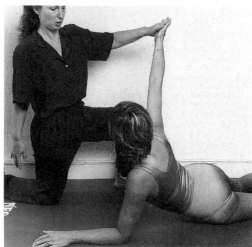

Fig. 4.3

Tests for Balance Reactions—*contd.*

Patient sitting on the plinth, his feet unsupported.

	Yes?	No?
a. He is pushed towards the affected side. Does he stay upright?		
Does he laterally flex his head towards the sound side?		
Does he abduct his sound leg?		
Does he use the affected forearm for support?		
Does he use the affected hand for support? (Fig. 4.4) . . .		
b. He is pushed forward. Does he bend affected hip and knee?		
Does he extend his spine?		
Does he lift his head? (Fig. 4.5)		

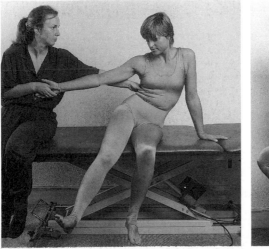

Fig. 4.4

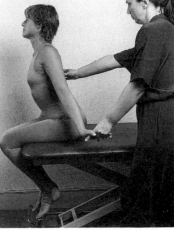

Fig. 4.5

Tests for Balance Reactions—*contd.*

	Yes?	No?
c. Both his legs are lifted up by the therapist, knees flexed. Does he stay upright?		
Does he move affected arm forward? (Fig. 4.6)		
Does he support himself backwards with affected arm?		

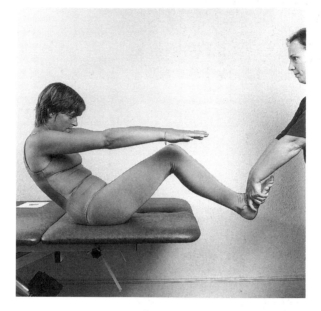

Fig. 4.6

Patient in four-foot kneeling	Yes?	No?
a. His body is pushed towards the affected side.		
Does he abduct the sound leg?		
Does he remain on all fours? (Fig. 4.7)		
b. His sound arm is lifted and held up by the therapist.		
Does he keep affected arm extended? (Fig. 4.8)		
c. His sound leg is lifted.		
Does he keep affected leg flexed and transfer weight on to it? (Fig. 4.9)		

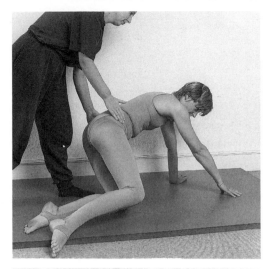

Fig. 4.7

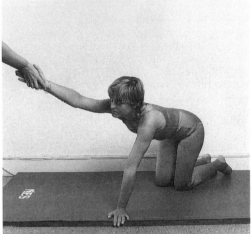

Fig. 4.8

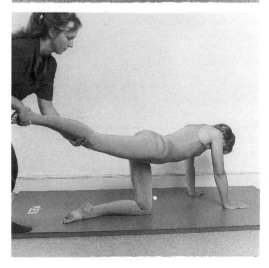

Fig. 4.9

Tests for Balance Reactions—*contd.*

	Yes?	No?
d. His sound arm and affected leg are lifted.		
Does he keep affected arm extended? (Fig. 4.10)		
e. His affected arm and his sound leg are lifted.		
Does he remain on affected flexed leg? (Fig. 4.11)		
f. His sound arm and leg are lifted.		
Does he transfer his weight towards the affected side and maintain position (Fig. 4.12)		

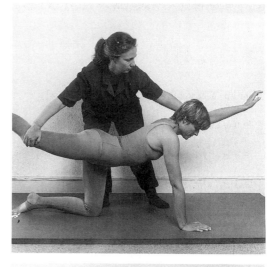

Fig. 4.10

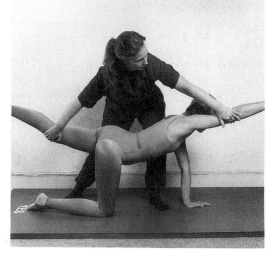

Fig. 4.11

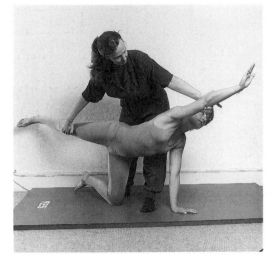

Fig. 4.12

Tests for Balance Reactions—*contd.*	Yes?	No?
Patient in kneel-standing.		
a. He is pushed towards the affected side.		
Does he abduct the sound leg?		
Does he bend head laterally towards the sound side? ...		
Does he use his affected hand for support? (Fig. 4.13) ..		
b. He is pushed towards the sound side.		
Does he abduct the affected leg?		
Does he extend the affected arm sideways? (Fig. 4.14) ..		
c. He is pushed backwards and asked not to sit down.		
Does he extend the affected arm forwards? (Fig. 4.15) ..		
d. He is pushed gently forwards, his sound arm held backwards by the therapist.		
Does he use affected arm and hand for support on the ground? (Fig. 4.16a)		
Does he lift affected foot off the ground? (Fig 4.16b)		

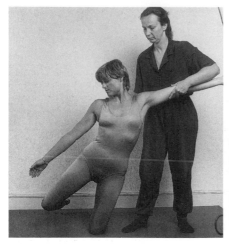

Fig. 4.13

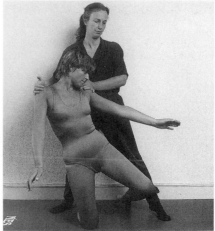

Fig. 4.14

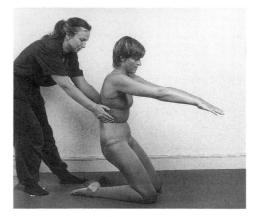

Fig. 4.15

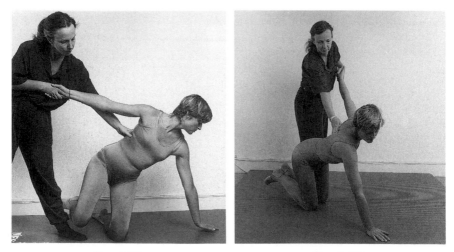

Fig. 4.16a

Fig. 4.16b

Tests for Balance Reactions—*contd.*

Patient half-kneeling, sound foot forwards. (He should not use sound hand for support.)

	Yes?	No?
a. His sound foot is lifted up by the therapist. Does he remain upright?		
Does he keep affected hip extended? (Fig. 4.17a)		
b. His sound foot is lifted by the therapist and placed sideways.		
Does he remain upright?		
Does he show balance movements with his affected arm? (Fig. 4.17b)		
c. His sound foot is placed from the above position back to kneel-standing.		
Does he keep upright?		
Does he keep affected hip extended?		

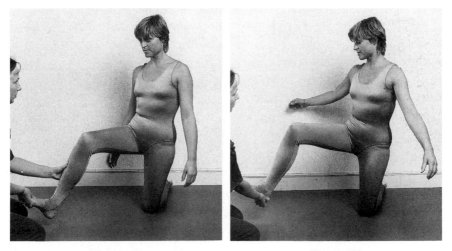

Fig. 4.17a   Fig. 4.17b

Tests for Balance Reactions—*contd.*

	Yes?	No?
Patient standing, feet parallel, standing base narrow.		
a. He is tipped backwards and not allowed to make step backwards with sound leg. (Therapist puts her foot on his sound one to prevent step.)		
Does he step backwards with affected leg? (Fig. 4.18) ..		
b. He is tipped backwards and not allowed to make steps with either leg.		
Does he dorsiflex toes of affected leg?		
Big toe only?		
Dorsiflex ankle and toes of affected leg?		
Does he move affected arm forwards? (Fig. 4.19)		
c. He is tipped towards sound side.		
Does he abduct affected leg?		
Does he abduct and extend affected arm? (Fig. 4.20a) ..		
Does he make steps to follow with affected leg across sound leg? (Fig. 4.20b)		

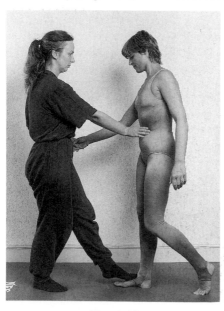

Fig. 4.18

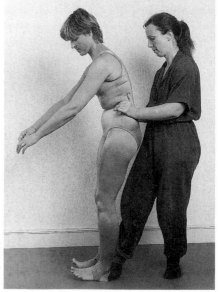

Fig. 4.19

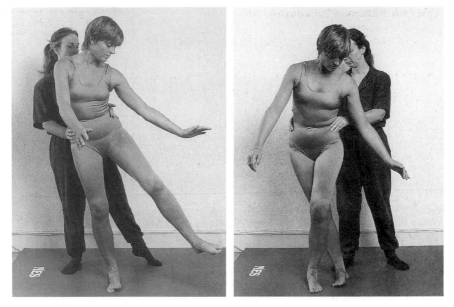

Fig. 4.20a   Fig. 4.20b

Tests for Balance Reactions—*contd.*

d. He is tipped towards the affected side.

Does he abduct the sound leg? . . . .

Does he bend head laterally towards the sound side? . . .
(Fig. 4.21)

	Yes?	No?

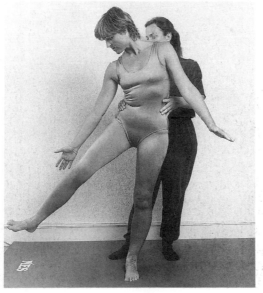

Fig. 4.21

Tests for Balance Reactions—*contd.*

	Yes?	No?

Patient standing on affected leg only. (He is not allowed to use sound hand for support.)

a. His sound foot is lifted by the therapist and moved forwards as in making a step, extending his knee.

Does he keep the heel of affected leg on the ground? . . . .

Does he keep the knee of the affected leg extended? . . . . .

Does he assist weight transfer forward over affected leg with extended hip? (Fig. 4.22) . . . .

b. His sound foot is lifted by the therapist and moved backwards as in making a step backwards.

Does he keep the hip of affected leg extended? . . . .

Does he assist weight transfer backwards over affected leg? (Fig. 4.23) . . . .

c. His sound foot is lifted by the therapist and held up while he is *pushed* gently sideways towards the affected side.

Does he follow and adjust his balance, moving the foot of the affected leg sideways by inverting and everting his foot alternately? . . . .

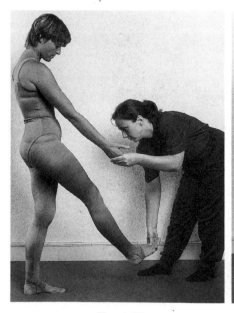

Fig. 4.22

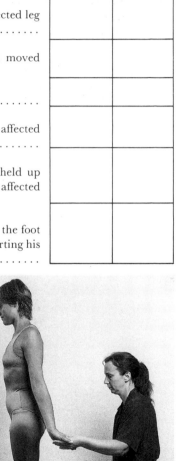

Fig. 4.23

Tests for Balance Reactions—*contd.*

	Yes?	No?
The same manoeuvre is done *pulling* him towards the affected side.		
Does he follow and adjust his balance by moving his foot as above?		

2. Tests for Protective Extension and Support of the Arm

When testing these reactions the patient's sound arm should be held by his hand so that he cannot use it. It is advisable to hold the sound arm in extension and external rotation because this facilitates the extension of the affected arm and hand.

	Yes?	No?
a. The patient stands in front of a table or plinth. His sound arm is held backwards and he is pushed forwards towards the table.		
Does he extend his affected arm forward?		
Does he support himself on his fist?		
On the palm of his hand? (Fig. 4.24)		
His thumb adducted?		
His thumb abducted? (Fig. 4.24)		

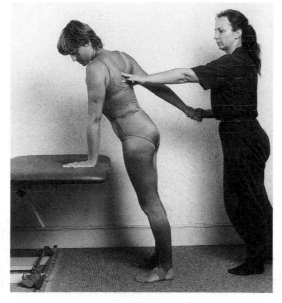

Fig. 4.24

Tests for Protective Extension and Support of the Arm—*contd.*

	Yes?	No?
b. The patient stands facing a wall, at a distance which allows him to reach it with his hand. He is pushed forward against the wall, his sound arm held backwards.		
Does he lift his affected arm and stretch it out against the wall?		
Does he place his hand against the wall, fingers flexed, thumb adducted?		
Fingers open, thumb abducted? (Fig. 4.25)		
c. The patient is sitting on the plinth. His sound arm is held sideways by the therapist. He is pushed towards the affected side.		
Does he abduct the affected arm and support himself on his forearm?		
On his extended arm?		
Does he support himself on his fist?		
On his open palm?		
Thumb and fingers adducted?		
Thumb and fingers abducted? (Fig. 4.4)		
d. The patient stands sideways to a wall, at a distance which allows him to reach it with his affected hand.		
Does he abduct and lift the affected arm?		
With flexed elbow?		
Does he reach out for the wall with extended elbow? . . .		
Does he support himself with his fist against the wall? . .		
With his open hand?		
With adducted thumb and fingers?		
With abducted thumb and fingers? (Fig. 4.26)		

Tests for Protective Extension and Support of the Arm—*contd.*

	Yes?	No?
e. The patient lies on the floor on his back. His sound hand is placed under his hip so that he cannot use it. The therapist takes a pillow and pretends to throw it towards his head.		
Does he move his affected arm to protect his face?		
With flexed elbow?		
With extended elbow?		
With internal rotation?		
With external rotation?		
With fisted hand?		
With open hand?		
Can he catch the pillow? (Fig. 4.27)		

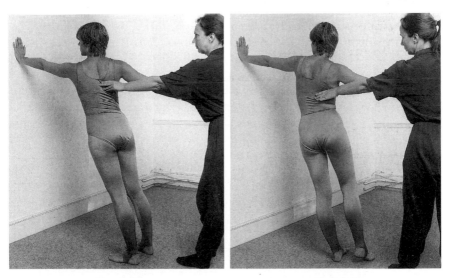

Fig. 4.25   Fig. 4.26

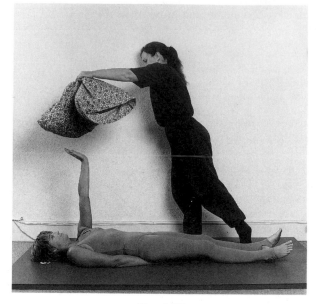

Fig. 4.27

SUMMARY

The foregoing suggested tests should be used during treatment as well as for initial assessment of the patient's needs. They are not intended to be used as a 'test battery' on every patient, one test after another before treatment is begun. Testing in this way gives the therapist not only constant information about the patient's ability and disability and about improvement achieved or not achieved, but it also gives a guide for necessary changes of treatment and for the way in which treatment should be progressed.

The importance of a close link between assessment and treatment has been presented, together with three groups of detailed tests specifically designed to assess the hemiplegic patient's motor patterns. The results of the tests will give the therapist a guide to the planning of treatment and information on the patient's progress.

5

THE CONCEPT AND PRINCIPLES OF TREATMENT

The usual aim of treatment during the early and acute stage of adult hemiplegia is that of short-term rehabilitation with a view to getting the patient out of bed and making him as independent as possible in the activities of daily living. In order to get him to walk as soon as possible, the emphasis in treatment is placed on the sound side in compensation for loss of the affected side. He is given a tripod on which to lean, which brings his whole weight towards the sound side and makes him use his sound leg for balance and walking. As he cannot bend his knee and ankle, he has to use his trunk to help him to bring the affected leg forward to make a step, causing him to 'hitch' up his pelvis. The leg is stiff and is used momentarily as a prop to carry his weight, most of which is taken on the tripod or elbow crutch or, later on, on a stick. The patient is taught, also, to use his sound arm and hand for self-help, for pushing or pulling himself up to sitting, for getting out of bed, for standing up from a chair, etc. This programme of 'compensatory rehabilitation' is usually supplemented with exercises to strengthen muscles and to maintain joint ranges. The two, however, are given as separate procedures. They have little to do with each other and are, in fact, mutually exclusive, as rehabilitation by compensation is to a large extent responsible for an increase in spasticity and for the inactivity of the involved side.

It may be argued that such short-term rehabilitation in hospital saves time and has economical advantages. However, even after discharge from hospital the patient needs further treatment for a prolonged period in the outpatient department or at home. If the potential recovery of the affected side and its treatment is taken into consideration from the beginning and throughout the whole time of the patient's treatment, his rehabilitation will not take longer and the results will be better.

It is regrettable if treatment neglects the potentialities of the affected side right from the start and is especially regrettable in the case of patients who are still young enough to lead a useful life. In fact, such treatment in the acute case makes subsequent restoration of function of the affected limbs during the residual stage, i.e. when outpatient treatment is given, more difficult and even impossible for, by this time, over-compensation with a more than necessary use of the sound side has become firmly established; spasticity is very strong due to associated reactions caused by the effort needed for unilateral use of the sound side, and also through lack of balance and fear of falling.

Our experience has shown that is is possible to get a great deal of normal activity out of the affected side by a treatment which is systematically designed to prepare the affected side for functional use. It has even been found possible to improve gait and balance, and the use of the arm in many patients with longstanding residual hemiplegia, although function of the hand has been found possible only in those patients who had no, or little sensory deficit. This experience proved that there had been an unsuspected and untapped potential which short-term compensatory rehabilitation did not touch. Quicker and better results could be obtained if, during the early stage while the patient is still in hospital, the emphasis in treatment is planned on developing the functional potentialities of the affected side, instead of writing it off as useless.

The patient's main problem is his inability to direct the nervous impulses to his muscles in the many varied ways and in the different combinations of patterns used by a person with an intact central nervous system. The main task of treatment is that of improving tonus and coordination by obtaining normal active reactions of the affected side in response to being moved. Normal reactions to being moved indicate the patient's ability to perform the same movements independently and voluntarily.

The patient's more normal reactions to being moved during treatment show us his potential and are a guide to the therapist in planning treatment. They also show which techniques to use and not to use, and how to use them, all this depending on the patient's responses throughout the treatment. It is important to monitor these responses for better or worse by a constant feed-back between patient and therapist. If in doubt about whether a response is normal or not, the therapist can and should do the same manoeuvre on the patient's sound side for comparison.

The aim of treatment should be to inhibit the patient's abnormal patterns of movement because we cannot superimpose normal on abnormal patterns. They should not be reinforced and perpetuated by the effort involved in strengthening the muscles. The movements the patient performs with or without the therapist's help should not be done with undue effort. Effort leads to an increase of spasticity and produces widespread associated reactions.

Heavy resistance exercises (Walters, 1967), irradiation (Knott, 1967), and the use of associated reactions and mass synergies (Brunnstrom, 1956 a, b) may be useful in strengthening weak and unresponsive muscles in orthopaedic cases and in patients with lower motor neurone problems. However, they should be avoided in patients with upper motor neurone lesions, i.e. when tonic reflexes are disinhibited and dominant to the total, or almost total, exclusion of every other pattern of coordination. The influence of tonic reflexes is present in normal persons and produces slight and transient tonus changes among the wealth of many other postural and movement patterns. But in spastic conditions, if disinhibited, the use of effort, irradiation, and of the mass patterns of tonic reflexes to strengthen muscles, will only reinforce the existing released tonic reflexes and, with it, increase spasticity.

In the patient with spasticity, more normal coordination cannot be obtained as long as released tonic reflexes are active, evidenced by the abnormal postural patterns of extensor and flexor spasticity. As mentioned before, spasticity is not confined to any one muscle or muscle group, but is coordinated in definite synergic patterns. Their inhibition reduces spasticity and this can be done by the therapist changing and dissociating the spastic patterns, i.e. by 'shunting' (*see* p. 18). However, without the patient being active while the therapist changes a position, there is no carry-over of this inhibitory action into his own and unassisted movement. The patient has to learn to control actively the widespread total patterns of spasticity.

It has been found ineffective to use static reflex-inhibiting patterns, the original reflex-inhibiting 'postures'. Although spasticity becomes reduced temporarily, there is no carry-over into the patient's own functional activity. If he attempts to move independently, spasticity returns immediately, as he can only use the total spastic patterns. The therapist has to help him to use only parts of the total pattern and prevent the reassertion by her handling. The patient is encouraged and enabled to use parts of the total pattern selectively. While he moves, the therapist prevents, i.e. inhibits, the unwanted parts of the abnormal total pattern. It is the restoration of this inhibitory control that makes the permanent reduction of spasticity possible, and gives him selective movements and their various combinations of functional skills. By learning to inhibit unwanted spread of activity throughout the affected parts of his body, he controls associated reactions. We may call this process 'autoinhibition'.

Two examples of obtaining and increasing the patient's inhibitory control of his spasticity are as follows:

1.   A patient with a severe degree of spasticity of the arm and hand, when sitting, is asked to move his trunk slowly towards the sound side and then forwards and backwards as far as possible. While he moves in this way, the therapist holds his affected hand fully extended at wrist and fingers, the arm in external rotation. The movements are done entirely by the patient and not by the therapist, who only follows the patient's movements while she gives inhibition distally: the patient needs only to move as far in any direction as is acceptable and comfortable for him. He is in control of the ranges of movements and confident that he can stop whenever he is uncomfortable. Treatment done in this way

is more effective in reducing severe degrees of spasticity than when the therapist moves the patient's arm against his trunk (Figs. 5.1a–f).

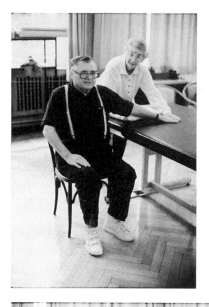

Fig. 5.1 *Patient moves trunk against arm and hand to inhibit flexor spasticity. (a) initial position; (b) trunk moves towards arm; (c) trunk moves away from arm; (d) trunk moves sideways from arm; (e) trunk moves forward. Therapist controls hand; (f) therapist does not control hand any longer.*

(a)

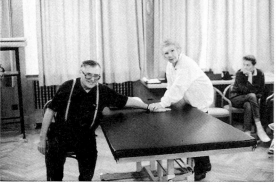

(b)

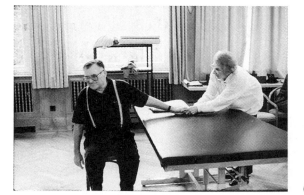

(c)

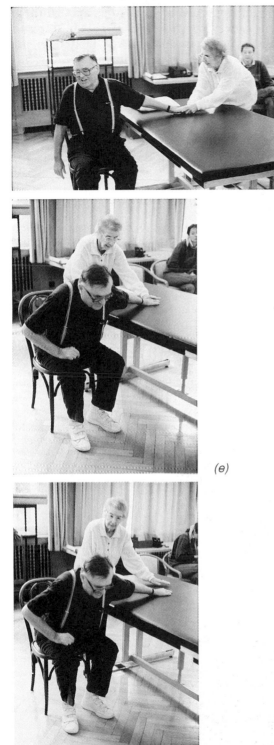

(d)

(e)

(f)

2.   Many patients with flexor spasticity of the arm find it uncomfortable when the arm bends and rides up in standing and walking. The patient can learn to control this flexion in the following way: he starts by sitting on a chair and bending his trunk forward and downward so that his arms hang down and extend at the elbows (Fig. 5.2a). He then moves and swings his affected arm (Fig. 5.2b) which is followed by swinging both arms. Then he slowly raises his trunk to sitting up straight. He keeps his head bent down to begin with while his arm remains hanging down, extended at the elbow, and lastly he raises his head slowly to stand up and walk (Fig. 5.2c). When the elbow flexes again, he repeats the movement forward downwards with his trunk until the elbow extends again (Figs. 5.2d–f).*

It is interesting and necessary for the therapist to find out at which stage of the patient's walking, the arm flexes again. It may be when he makes a step with the sound leg, which shows he has insufficient weightbearing and balance on the affected one, or when he steps with the affected leg, which indicates that extensor spasticity makes it difficult for him to lift it for a step. Treatment has then to take these findings into account.

Twitchell (1951) describes the absence of spasticity when isolated movements become possible. It appears, therefore, that the reduction

* More examples of autoinhibition are given on pp. 151–156.

Fig. 5.2   Autoinhibition of flexor spasticity of arm. (a) swinging both arms, elbow extended; (b) slowly raising trunk, elbow extended; (c) slowly standing up; (d) when elbow flexes, patient bends down again; (e) keeping elbow extended when standing up; (f) walking, keeping elbow extended.

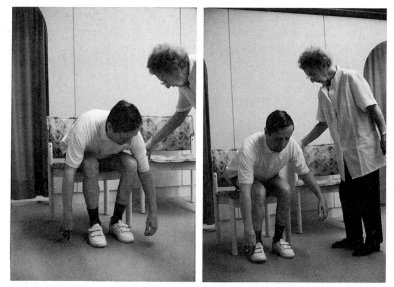

(a)   (b)

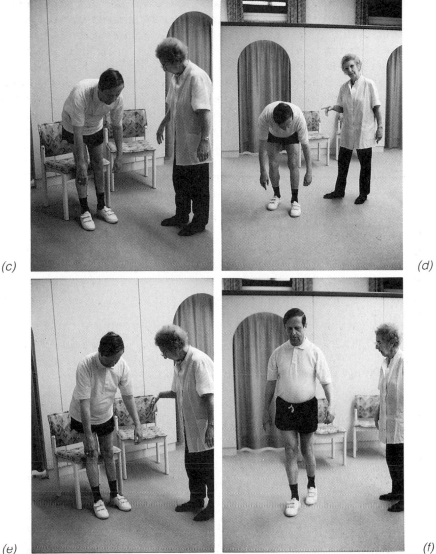

(c)

(d)

(e)

(f)

of spasticity in treatment makes isolated movements possible, or, that isolated movements reduce spasticity. In treatment, the first selective movements can usually be obtained at elbow and knee through weightbearing on arm or leg, as this makes the necessary fixation for an isolated movement easier to obtain. Selective movement when not weightbearing, i.e. with less fixation, for instance, isolated movements of wrist and fingers, or of the elbow while lifting and holding the arm up, is much more difficult. Then the patient has to give proximal fixation to hold the limb up against gravity, while moving distal parts of it independently.

At later stages of recovery, and in patients with slight spasticity, treatment has to be advanced towards a further breaking up of patterns, obtaining the great variety of selective movements needed for functional skills. In this way, the patient's inhibitory control increases and, with it, his threshold to stimulation is gradually increased. Inhibition of unwanted patterns of function is part and parcel of every treatment. An example of the many ways in which it can be used is, for instance, the clasping of hands while lifting and moving the extended arm, the movement being controlled by the patient's sound arm and hand. In this way he inhibits the spastic pattern of flexion, pronation, adduction of the fingers and internal rotation of the arm at the shoulder and thus reduces spasticity.

The exercising of 'autoinhibition' is not only beneficial for one specific movement, but, by reducing spasticity generally, it also gives control over other movements.

Treatment has become more active and dynamic. Instead of *static postures*, reflex inhibiting *movement* patterns are used which not only inhibit abnormal postural reactions, but, at the same time facilitate active automatic and voluntary movements. *Inhibition facilitates and facilitation inhibits.* With the help of reflex inhibiting movements, the output from the CNS is directed (shunted) into more normal patterns of activity while inhibiting abnormal motor patterns. Instead of reversing the spastic patterns in their totality, the therapist can reduce spasticity throughout all the affected parts of the body by changing only parts of the abnormal pattern. These are called *key points* of control. The dissociation of the total patterns of spasticity serves not only to obtain voluntary and selective movements, but also gives the patient control over whole sequences of both voluntary and automatic movements. The most important key points are proximal, but there are also distal key points.

Proximal key points are the trunk, i.e. the spine with its connections to the head, shoulder and pelvic girdles. From there, we can influence tonus and movements distally. The patterns of spasticity show a combination of both total patterns of flexor and extensor hypertonus. The patient cannot combine parts of a flexor pattern with parts of an extensor pattern as in normal functional activity. Rotation between pelvis and shouldergirdle or vice versa plays an important role in the dissociation of the total patterns of both flexion and extension. Distal key points are part of a limb, e.g. elbow, knee, hands and feet. They influence tonus and movements proximally, so that the trunk and head can be left free to move actively for righting and balance. Both types of key points are used in combination because their effect on tonus and movement overlaps. The use of proximal key points facilitates movements of the limbs while distal key points facilitate movements of the trunk.

Key points are interchangeable and have to be adapted to the patient's reactions. The control of sequences of movements needs the changing of key points while the patient moves, and according to which patterns the therapist wishes to inhibit or facilitate during the movement. Therefore, no one key point can be made responsible, or can be used, for obtaining whole sequences of movement. The therapist, by using key points, facilitates not only a different pattern, but gives the necessary fixation for independent movement elsewhere. It is essential for the therapist to withdraw her control gradually while the movement proceeds, because her control interferes with the patient's ability to be active where she controls. His own control is only possible where and when he is left free to move without her interference. Autoinhibition enables the patient to gain control over his spasticity. When the therapist has made it possible for him to inhibit the abnormal patterns of spasticity, his movements become more normally coordinated and, by themselves, then reduce spasticity.

The main reflex inhibiting patterns counteracting flexor spasticity in the trunk and arm is extension of neck and spine and external rotation of the arm and shoulder with extended elbow. Further reduction of flexor spasticity can be obtained by adding extension of the wrist with supination and abduction of the thumb. The fact that extension of the flexor-spastic arm occurs when the patient is in supine and his arm is elevated does not mean that there is inhibition of flexor spasticity, but only a change of the pattern of flexor spasticity in favour of extensor spasticity. Then flexion of the elbow is resisted and the patient cannot touch his face or the top of his head. Similarly, if the patient bends down and forward with his trunk, the arm extends at the elbow and he cannot bend it to bring his hand to his face. This phenomenon was described by Russel Brain (1927) and called by him the 'quadrupedal extension reflex'.

In both instances, flexor spasticity is not inhibited; there has been only a change of one spastic pattern for another, neither being of functional use. The main reflex inhibiting pattern which counteracts both extensor and flexor spasticity of the leg is abduction with external rotation and extension of hip and knee. Further reduction of extensor spasticity can be obtained by adding dorsiflexion of toes and ankle with abduction of the big toe. Another important reflex inhibiting pattern is rotation of the shouldergirdle against the pelvis and, more importantly, of the pelvis against the shouldergirdle.

These are but a few examples of a great many reflex inhibiting patterns which can be used to reduce spasticity. They have to be adapted and varied to each individual patient's abnormal postural reactions. Reflex-inhibiting patterns not only inhibit abnormal activity but, at the same time, they give the patient normal 'postural sets' to initiate movements.

The inhibition of abnormal postural reflex activity is immediately combined with the activation of the patient. He may be asked to do a certain movement such as standing up or sitting down, turning over, reaching out, etc., while the therapist controls his postural reactions and tonus from key points only. Or — without asking him for a voluntary movement — he may be handled and moved with special techniques of facilitation which call for automatic adjustment of his posture, that is for active movements, such as balance and other protective reactions. In the normal person the required 'postural sets' which make movements easy and economical are automatic. For instance, if we turn the head to look behind us we first rotate the shouldergirdle. If we want to get up from a chair, we first adjust our legs and trunk to stand up. Due to his condition, the hemiplegic patient is confined to a static 'postural set', which prevents all other movements that do not belong to it. In order to make these movements possible, the patient should be given postural sets which facilitate them instead of blocking them. Facilitation techniques are designed to obtain specific normal movements in response to special ways of handling the patient.

These postural sets, i.e. adaptations of posture, change with the intended movement — in fact, they may precede it. Horak (1987) says:

> 'Postural adjustments occur not only as a result of sensory feedback in response to unexpected, external perturbations, but also as a result of 'feedback' in anticipation of expected self-generated perturbations.'

From the beginning of treatment the patient with spasticity has to learn to use his muscles in many different ways and in many combinations of patterns, and he can only do this while spasticity has been reduced. As therapists, we have to enable him to experience the normal sensations of functional movements which he has lost, for only by 'feeling' a normal movement with normal effort, which is minimal, can he again 'learn' how it is done. The hemiplegic patient, like a normal person, does not learn movements, but the 'sensation' of movements. The sensory experiences of the patient, however, are those resulting from the spastic condition of his muscles. He *feels* the excessive effort when trying to move. His limbs feel heavy, but in spite of his efforts, he feels too weak to move them. He experiences only the sensation of one posture and very restricted ranges of movement of his joints. It is essential in treatment to give the patient as many sensations of normal tone, posture and movement as possible. The therapist has, therefore, to help him with her hands to experience the sensation of different and more normal postures and movements against the background of a more normal postural tone.

Generally speaking, the patient with slight or moderate spasticity is not too 'weak' to move. Lack of muscle power may not be due to weakness, but to the opposition of spastic antagonists. If the latter's spasticity is reduced, the seemingly weak muscles may contract effectively. Drachman (1967) writes: 'Increased tone may interfere with normal movement to a degree far out of proportion to the underlying weakness.' In the patient with spasticity, contraction of a muscle does not result in reciprocal inhibition of its antagonist, because there is excessive co-contraction, a typical feature of spasticity. Therefore, reciprocal inhibition of spastic antagonists by activating a prime mover cannot be relied on in the treatment of spastic patients.

From the foregoing, it will be seen that the main problem in patients with upper motor neurone lesions is twofold: (1) abnormal coordination and (2) abnormal postural tone. Two main aims, namely (1) the reduction of spasticity and (2) the introduction of more selective movement patterns, both automatic and voluntary, in preparation for functional skills, should be followed in treatment. The carry-over of treatment, that is, the permanent reduction of spasticity, is only obtained when the patient is able to perform selective movements actively. This has been observed by Twitchell (1951) who says:

> 'The next event in recovery of movement was the occurrence of ability to flex either shoulder, elbow, all the fingers or wrist, each without the other. This separation of the elements of a synergic complex was only gradually achieved . . . If power and dexterity of voluntary movement continued to improve, a stage was reached where spasticity abruptly lessened, first in the shoulder and elbow muscles, and later in the flexors of wrist and fingers.'

In the patient with flaccidity or *real* weakness of muscles, postural activity has to be increased and this is achieved by using tactile and proprioceptive stimulation. However, in these patients all techniques of stimulation have to be used with great care, as they may result in abnormal tonic reflex activity instead of producing normal increase of postural tone and normal coordination of muscle action. This can be avoided by carefully grading stimulation and by using reflex inhibiting patterns simultaneously with techniques of stimulation, so that the patient's motor output in response to sensory input can be controlled and remain normal.

It is most important to plan treatment on the basis of a good assessment of the individual patient's needs. This should include assessment of:

1. his postural tone and changes of tone under conditions of stimulation in different positions and movements;
2. the quality of his postural and movement patterns, and
3. his functional abilities and disabilities.

A treatment plan is then made, stating the general aims of treatment, as, for instance:

1. whether to decrease, increase, or stabilize postural tone;
2. which postural patterns or movement reactions should be inhibited and which should be obtained and facilitated;
3. which are the functional skills for which the patient should be prepared, in what order and with which methods.

The choice of the actual patterns and techniques of treatment to be employed in the individual case of certain stages of treatment are derived from the general assessment.

6

TECHNIQUES OF TREATMENT

The many ways of treatment described in this chapter are intended to be suggestions and ideas of what can be done with a patient. They should *not* be regarded as a succession of exercises or patterns to be used, in the order given, for *all* patients. It must always be remembered that the aim of this type of treatment is to improve the quality of movement on the affected side, so that ultimately the two sides work together as harmoniously as possible within the scope of the cerebral injury. The techniques which a therapist may choose to use from among the many given will depend, therefore, on what the individual patient needs first and foremost to set him on the road to as near normal a recovery as possible. The chosen techniques must then be tried out with the patient and their effect tested within the same treatment session. The effect, whether good or bad, will show itself in changes in the patient's postural tone, motor patterns and functional use, as a continual response to the therapist's handling. No one pattern and no one technique should be made responsible for an expected reaction. If no change can be observed, or if there is a change for the worse, the attempted procedure must be discontinued. However, it may not necessarily be the technique or the pattern which is unsuitable: it may be the way it is used which fails to produce the desired response. There is a great deal of experimentation involved in good treatment, and everything depends on the constant feed-back between patient and therapist. Techniques are tools and are, therefore, interchangeable. We treat the 'reactions' of the patient and are constantly guided by his response to our handling. This kind of treatment reveals to the therapist, during the actual process of treatment, the effects which are taking place, and thus enables her to know which of the many techniques she may be using is responsible for improvement and which are harmful or useless. All too often certain techniques are used for long periods of time in the hope that one day they will produce results, even though no improvement can be noticed during any treatment session. The constant adjustment of the techniques to the response of the patient will not only prevent waste of time, but will make possible a more systematic treatment and give better results. Further, it will give indications as to what has been useful in any one particular type of patient and point the way to what may be equally useful and successful in other patients, who show similar difficulties and needs.

The techniques employed depend on the stage of recovery the patient has reached, or at which the process of recovery has become arrested. These stages may be defined as:

1. Initial flaccid stage.
2. Stage of spasticity.
3. Stage of relative recovery.

The recovery of the individual patient may be arrested at any one of these stages. If treatment cannot be given immediately after the onset of hemiplegia, it has to be started at the stage of recovery the patient has reached. Moreover, it should be borne in mind that the three stages overlap and cannot be clearly separated. Some degree of spasticity may already be found during the flaccid stage, or the patient may have some fairly independent movement of the limbs during the spastic stage. Furthermore, even during the third stage of relative recovery, spasticity may still interfere with selective movements when the patient has to use effort for a more difficult task.

THE INITIAL FLACCID STAGE

A stroke produces a complete and sudden change and the patient has no time to adjust himself to it gradually. He is confused and disorientated, and the two sides of his body present him with different sensations. He is, so to speak, divided into two halves and there is no interplay whatever between the sound and the affected sides. As there is no balance or arm support on the affected side, the patient has a great fear of falling towards that side, which increases spasticity — even normal people become stiff when they are afraid of falling. All this leads to the negation of the affected side by the patient and to a complete orientation towards the sound side, an effect which should be counteracted in treatment and not reinforced.

Treatment started in the early stages should help the patient to carry weight on the affected side and to learn to balance on that side in sitting and standing. It should also help in working for bilateral function of arms and trunk, so that the required interplay of the sound side with the affected side becomes possible.

The initial flaccid stage is found soon after the onset of hemiplegia and lasts from a few days to several weeks and may be longer. The patient cannot move his affected side and often does not appreciate that he has an arm or a leg on that side. He has lost his former patterns of movement and, at first, even those of his sound side are inadequate to compensate for the loss of activity on the affected side. He now has to use his sound side in a different way and does not know immediately how to do this. At this stage, there is no restriction of joint range to passive movements on the affected side. Though there may not, as yet, be signs of spasticity, retraction of the scapula may be found with some resistance to passive movement of the shouldergirdle forward. Fingers and wrist may be slightly flexed and, on quick passive extension, some resistance may be felt. There may also be slight resistance to full supination of the forearm and wrist when this is done with the elbow extended. The first signs of spasticity may be felt when dorsiflexing the ankle and toes with the hip and knee in extension, and in some cases there may be slight resistance to pronation of the foot.

The patient's position in bed is as follows: the neck usually shows slight lateral flexion towards the affected side, the shoulder and arm are retracted and the elbow still extended at this stage. The forearm is pronated.* The leg is usually extended and laterally rotated, the ankle plantiflexed and often slightly supinated.‡ A few patients, usually the very old or the severely affected ones, lie with a flexed and abducted leg and supinated foot. In all cases, the whole of the affected side, i.e. shoulder and pelvis, is slightly rotated backwards.

The patient cannot turn over towards the sound side, cannot sit unsupported and cannot stand or walk. He tends to fall towards the affected side as he has no mid-line orientation. This latter is an interesting phenomenon in that normally the activity of the sound side would prevent him from falling to the affected side. It may be explained by the fact that the sound side does not 'know' what is happening on the affected side, as there is no interplay between them and the sensations on each side are completely different.

As long as there is only lack of tonus and no spasticity, there will be no associated reactions on moving the sound limbs.

Nursing as Preparation for Turning Over, Sitting Up, Standing and Walking

In the early stages, the nursing staff have an important role to play in the rehabilitation of the patient, especially while he is still bed- or chair-bound and in need of a great deal of nursing care. At this time, it is possible to make many mistakes in the way in which the patient is handled, which could have an unfavourable effect on the future chances of treatment and rehabilitation. By adequate positioning and handling of the patient, an undue increase of spasticity can be prevented, as can contractures, shoulder pain and shoulder-hand syndrome, retraction of shouldergirdle and pelvis, and even the rejection of the affected side.

Physiotherapy and nursing should be complementary to one another since physiotherapy and nursing care overlap. In this early stage, the nursing staff care for the patient all day long, while the

* Pronation equals eversion of the foot.
‡ Supination equals inversion of the foot.

physiotherapist is with him for only a short time each day. The physiotherapist teaches the patient how to move again, while the nursing staff can be shown how to help the patient towards the ultimate goals and achievements of treatment by the way in which they position and handle him in the early stage. The physiotherapist and the occupational therapist can, in their turn, help the nurses by getting the patient to gain some independence and thus lighten their burden.

Cooperation Between Nurses and Therapists

Cooperation is, therefore, not only desirable, but also vital. It can be achieved by good communication between the different ancillary services and by nurses understanding the special problems of the hemiplegic patient. These problems are not only different from those of patients without cerebral injury, but also differ from one hemiplegic to another. Many problems are similar in all hemiplegics, but not all are affected to the same extent or in the same way. Sensory deficits of varying degrees, different tonus qualities, the patient's age, his anxiety and insecurity, confusion, mental and emotional state and speech involvement, all cause different individual problems. The patient's condition changes with treatment and often remits spontaneously. As his abilities develop, different problems are encountered. By giving help and support to certain parts of his body, the therapist and nurse enable the patient to take an active part when he is being helped to move, and by this means he learns how to move unaided. At first, the patient can perform only parts of a movement sequence e.g. partially turn over in bed, partially sit up, partially stand up from sitting on the bed or chair, etc. He has to re-learn all his movements, often even on the unaffected side, because now the sound side has to be used differently to adapt itself to the loss of use on the affected side. The patient cannot learn this quickly, nor can he actively follow quick movements done with him by his therapist. He has to be given sufficient time to cooperate when he is being moved, and much repetition of the same movements is needed. It happens all too frequently that the patient is moved too quickly and without his active cooperation. At this same time, many patients are expected to dress themselves, get up, walk and become independent as quickly as possible, without any gradual and systematic preparation to help them to achieve this independence.

The nurse's handling of the patient should not differ from the way he is handled by the physiotherapist in this early stage. If there were a marked difference, the patient would not be able to establish any newly learned movements nor could there be a carry-over into daily life.

To achieve good cooperation, the physiotherapist should inform the nurse from time to time about the progress the patient has made and what he has learned to do by himself or with a minimum of help. She should also show the nurse the way in which she handles the patient and what changes she has made in his treatment. It would be advantageous if the nurse, or sister, together with the physiotherapist, could make a first assessment of the patient's abilities and disabilities, and then also be present from time to time during physiotherapy sessions. This collaboration would enable the nursing staff to be much more involved in the actual rehabilitation of the patient, making their work more rewarding and less routine.

It is appreciated, however, that the nursing staff have their problems, although much depends on the individual hospital. Frequently, there are too few nurses: they are over-worked and always in a hurry, which prevents any active cooperation by the patient. He needs, however, to be as active as possible while being moved as a preparation for moving unaided later on. If he is handled by two nurses when his bed is being made or when he is moved to a chair, he is given no chance to help even if he wishes to do so. It would, therefore, be better for the patient if he were handled by only one nurse and encouraged to help her. This may take a little longer than when two nurses handle him together but, as far as the nursing staff is concerned, the end result would be the same, as the second nurse could attend to another patient.

If the patient has to be nursed at home, it is necessary to instruct a relative as to how to handle him in the way described in the section *Positioning and Moving of Hemiplegic Patients*, p. 76.

Special Nursing Problems of Hemiplegics

Apart from the purely medical aspects such as heart, breathing, circulation etc., there are special problems in the care of hemiplegics which concern the nurses and ought to be understood by them. They are as follows:

1. *The patient's body is seemingly divided into two halves*, the one having nothing to do with the other. The patient may not feel the affected arm or leg at all but, even if there is no, or little, sensory deficit, he receives abnormal sensations from his muscles and immobile joints. The psychological effects of this division show themselves in the way the patient looks away from the affected side and in his rejection of the affected arm and leg.

2. *The postural tone of the two sides is different*. At first, the patient is flaccid and seems too weak to move his arm or leg. In some cases this lasts for only a few days, in others for a longer duration. Flaccidity affects the arm more and for longer periods than the leg. Sooner or later spasticity develops and he becomes too stiff to move. It increases if the patient exerts himself, if he

becomes excited, if he wants to communicate, but cannot speak, and if he is afraid. Spasticity shows itself in definite abnormal patterns of posture, i.e. in flexion and retraction of the arm and in extension of the leg with backward rotation of the pelvis. If spasticity becomes severe, it can in time result in contractures. It always interferes with the patient's ability to move later on; for example, it may prevent him from bending his knee and putting his heel down when walking, or it may cause the foot to turn over at the ankle; he will be unable to lift his arm, extend his elbow and wrist, or to open his hand and fingers to grasp. By special ways of positioning the patient when he is in bed or sitting in a chair, the nursing staff can help to avoid the abnormal postural patterns from becoming established; this positioning will prevent the spastic patterns and help to maintain, and even extend, the patient's potential function.

3. *The patient no longer knows how to move.* He has to re-learn how to turn over in bed, how to sit up and lie down, how to stand up, stand and walk. The patient is confused and often does not know how to use his normal side to make up for the loss of movement of the affected side. He no longer 'knows' his affected side or how to use it. He has little or no balance and is in fear of falling towards that side. This fear of falling is one of the greatest problems, not only in the early stages but even more so later on, when he stands and walks. For this reason, the nurse, the therapists and the relatives of the patient should be by the affected side when helping him and not — as usually happens — by his sound side, as he can use this side himself unaided. By being on his affected side, the carer can help him to carry his full weight on it and improve his balance, whereas, if she stands by his sound side, she would be unable to help him if he should lose his balance and tend to fall. Every movement the nurse does with him is new to him. He has to learn to adjust himself and to cope with every new situation. As mentioned before, he cannot do this quickly and has, in fact, to get used to every 'stage' of the movement. He should not be moved hurriedly by the nurse, nor should he be passive when being moved from one position to another. He should be given time and opportunity actively to follow the movements done with him. The physiotherapist will find out when and where help and support is needed and, more important, where it is not. The nurse will find that the patient can often do more than she expects if he is given the necessary, but minimal, help at the right moment and at the right place.

4. *The preceding three points,* viz: a seemingly divided body, different postural tone on each side, ignorance of how to move, all combine to engender a fear of falling in the patient for a long

time, even after he is able to walk with the aid of a stick. The problems of balance can already be seen in lying and sitting. No weight is carried on the affected side in sitting and standing. The lateral flexion of neck and trunk towards the affected side, together with the patient's inability to support himself with his affected arm, make him tend to fall to that side.

Positioning and Moving of Hemiplegic Patients for Nurses and Therapists

Arm and head

Position in bed: patient lying on his back.

To prevent shoulder retraction: place outstretched arm alongside the body on a pillow somewhat higher than the trunk. Place outstretched hand on pillow or, better if possible, supinated against the outside of the pillow.
Important: Place the head laterally to the unaffected side, and the affected shoulder on the pillow as far forward as possible (Fig. 6.1a).

Pelvis and leg

N.B. Different positioning is needed for patients with or without extensor spasticity.

(a) Patients with flexor tendency of the leg and lack of extensor tone. These patients remain more flaccid than spastic for longer following a very bad stroke. Some cases of senility especially may lack bladder or sphincter control.

The flexor tendency is dangerous for rehabilitation. If the flexor pattern is allowed to become established and contractures develop, this type of patient will not have enough extensor tonus to enable him to get up, to stand or to walk. Therefore, the therapist must *prevent* flexor contractures of the hip and knee, pressure sores of the lower leg, and supination of the foot (Fig. 6.1b).

Position in bed: lying on back. A pillow or sandbag is placed under the pelvis on the affected side in order to lift the pelvis (to avoid pelvic retraction). The pillow must be long enough to give support to the lateral side of the thigh. This *prevents* external rotation of the leg, but it must not, however, go beyond the middle position, i.e. produce internal rotation (Fig. 6.1c). If too much extension or supination of the ankle results, a board may be placed against the foot to give dorsiflexion and pronation.

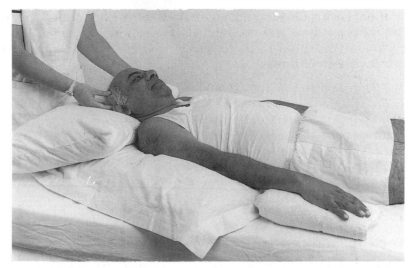

Fig. 6.1a   *Moving head laterally towards sound side, shoulder brought forward.*

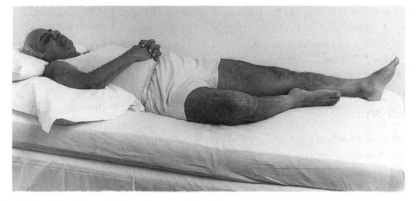

Fig. 6.1b   *Position of leg to be avoided.*
Note: *Flexion-abduction pattern of hip and knee and supination of foot.*

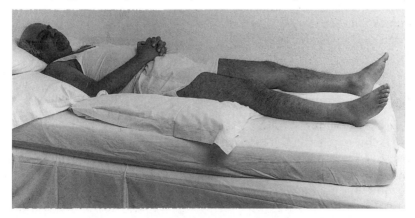

Fig. 6.1c   *Pelvis lifted and lateral aspect of thigh supported with pillow, resulting in good position of leg.*

(b) Patients who develop extensor spasticity early on. This will enable them to stand, but will impede flexion of the knee in walking. The patient tends to retract the pelvis and this produces excessive external rotation of the leg.

> *Position in bed:* the patient should not always be on his back, but should learn to lie on the sound and, also, the affected side. As in (a), support the pelvis and lift it forward with a sandbag or pillow. In order to avoid excessive extensor spasticity, the patient needs support under the knee by means of a small foam rubber cushion, with the knee slightly bent. No board should be placed against the foot, as he will push against it with his toes.

Movements in order to turn the patient over to his side

The following movements should first be practised in treatment with the physiotherapist and then be used by the nurses. Turning should commence with the upper part of the body and, in order to do this, the patient must first learn to lift the affected arm with the good arm, and to clasp his hands (i.e. with fingers interlocked). He should then lift his clasped hands, with elbows extended, to the horizontal and, if possible, above his head. From there, he should move his arms first to one side and then to the other (Fig. 6.2a). Turning over to the sound side should also be started with his arms and trunk, his hands clasped. He will then need only minimal help, if any, to turn his pelvis and move the affected leg to the sound side (Fig. 6.2b). When he is lying on the sound side, the shoulder of the affected side should be brought well forward, the arm supported on a pillow and extended at the elbow. The pillow can thus be 'embraced' by both arms. Turning over to the affected side is easier for the patient than turning to the sound side, and he may need no help at all, as he can use his sound arm and leg for turning over. When lying on the affected side, his involved shoulder should be brought well forward — the arm is then in external rotation and extended at the elbow (Fig. 6.2c).

Using the bedpan

The nurse will help him if necessary to bend the affected leg and place his foot flat on the bed. The patient will then bend the sound leg and place that foot parallel with and close to the affected foot. The nurse will fix both feet with one hand and ask the patient to lift his pelvis. She will then place the bedpan under the pelvis. The patient should keep his legs bent. If the affected foot does not remain in the initial position and slips away, the patient can fix it with the sound foot (Fig. 6.3a).

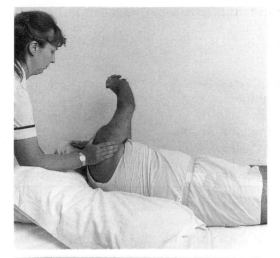

Fig.   6.2a With   hands
clasped,   turning   towards
sound side.
Note: *Movement started with
shoulder forward; knee kept in
slight flexion with small pillow.*

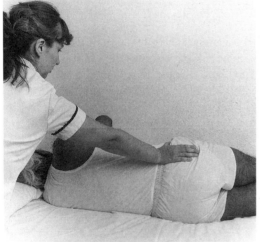

Fig.   6.2b Pelvis   moved
forward.

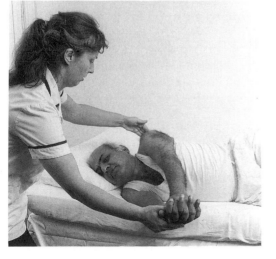

Fig. 6.2c Turning   towards
affected side, shoulder well
forward.

The patient pushes himself up in bed if he has slipped down

With help from the nurse, the patient follows through the first part of the movement described above when using the bedpan. His feet, which have been drawn up close to his pelvis, are held by the nurse who tells him to push himself upwards towards the head of the bed. The patient may find this difficult. The nurse should then fix his affected foot with one hand and help him up from the shoulder with her other hand. This is best done by placing her hand under his arm-pit, at the same time lifting the shoulder upwards and forwards, or she may lift his pelvis and help him in this way to push himself forwards (Figs. 6.3b, c).

Turning over to sit up on the side of the bed

(a) Turning to the sound side to sit up. As previously described (in *Turning Over* p. 78), the patient starts with clasped hands and supports himself on the sound forearm while he brings the sound leg over the edge of the bed into a half-sitting position. The nurse may help him to sit up by moving his head towards the affected side. At the same time, she moves the affected leg over the edge of the bed with her other hand. The patient should keep his hands clasped together (Fig. 6.4a). Some patients may not need the help of the nurse to lower the affected leg over the edge of the bed for sitting up if they have first been trained to move both legs flexed to one side or the other. With hands clasped, they start to turn the trunk and then the pelvis. The feet are on the bed and both knees are kept together when turning over. This is a good way of preparing the patient to move the affected leg over the edge of the bed (Figs. 6.4b, c).

(b) Turning to the affected side to sit up. This is somewhat more difficult for the patient, but it is necessary practice for him. The patient begins turning over as described above, i.e. with his hands clasped. When he is lying on the affected side and wants to sit up, the nurse supports his head on the affected side and helps him to move it towards his sound side and up, while he supports himself on the affected forearm. The nurse will help him to move the affected leg over the edge of the bed (Figs. 6.4d, e).

While the patient moves his sound leg over the edge of the bed, the nurse pushes his head further up from the affected side to the sound side and so to sitting up (Fig. 6.4f). If the patient's arm is not too spastic in flexion, she should place and hold the affected hand extended on the bed, so that the patient extends his elbow. During this phase, the sound arm is free to help the upward movement of the trunk.

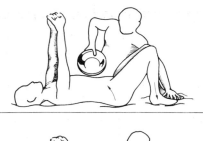

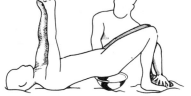

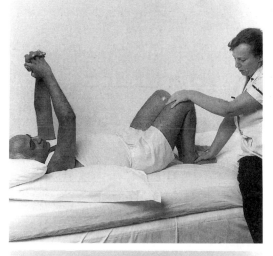

Fig. 6.3a   Patient lifts pelvis with feet fixed by therapist.

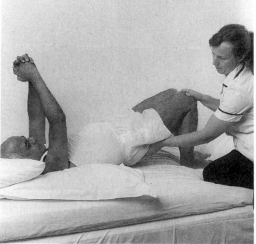

Fig. 6.3b   Fixing patient's foot with pressure down on flexed knee of hemiplegic leg, followed by—

Fig. 6.3c   Lifting pelvis to move patient upwards in bed.

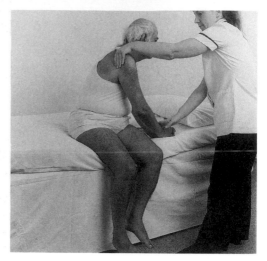

Fig. 6.4a Sitting up over the sound side.
Note: *Keep affected shoulder and arm well forward.*

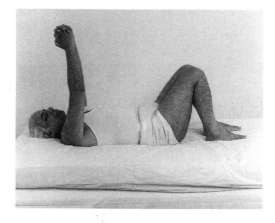

Figs. 6.4b, c Keeping knees together, patient turns to side-lying either side.

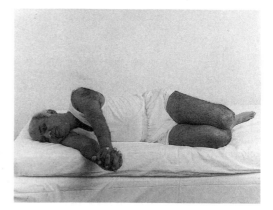

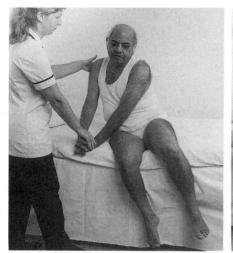

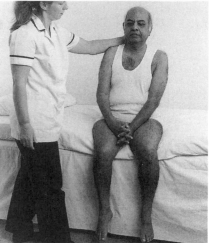

Fig. 6.4d Sitting up over the affected side.

Fig. 6.4e Therapist or nurse moves patient's head towards sound side.

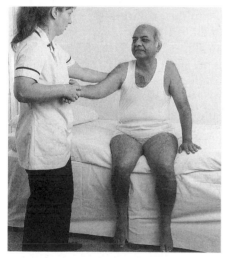

Fig. 6.4f Therapist moves shoulder and extended arm forward. Patient uses sound arm for support.

Lying down from sitting

The nurse holds the affected hand of the patient, his arm externally rotated and extended diagonally forward at shoulder height, while the patient slowly lies down, using his sound arm for support. In this way, the nurse will prevent retraction of the shoulder and flexion of the affected arm. The patient then lifts the sound leg on to the bed. If at all possible, he should then bend the affected leg at the knee and move it onto the bed, the nurse giving a little help by lifting from under the knee. He should not lift the affected leg with the sound one. This is in most cases unnecessary and is harmful, as the patient should not get into the habit of moving his leg passively with the sound one, but should learn to lift it actively as soon as possible.

Sitting and standing up

A foam rubber mat should be placed in front of the bed for standing. The nurse should never be on the patient's sound side when he sits, stands or walks, since he can use his sound side and does not need her there. She should stand either in front of him or, better still, at his affected side. This will enable her to shift his weight to the affected side in sitting, standing or walking, and in transferring to a chair or from a chair to the bed. If he takes weight on his affected side, the patient will gradually overcome his fear of falling.

Sitting up to stand. With the patient sitting on the bed, the nurse will stand in front of him and let him place his sound arm around her waist to hold on to her. She will then take the affected arm and, with one hand under his armpit, lift his shoulder, rotate the arm outwards and extend the elbow. Then she will bring the arm forward and against her waist just like the sound arm (Fig. 6.5a). She will fix his arm against her body with her forearm, so that both her hands will be free to help the patient to stand up. Before he stands up, she will help him to move forward from the hips, since he tends to retract his affected shoulder and lean his trunk backwards, especially on the affected side (Fig. 6.5b). Usually, the patient is afraid of falling even if someone is standing in front of him. He is also afraid of falling to the affected side. This fear can be alleviated by the nurse placing one of her hands under his shoulder and holding on to it while drawing him lightly towards the affected side, so that his weight is brought to bear on the affected hip. She can use her other hand to push his head sideways towards the sound side, as falling towards the affected side usually originates from the head. This lateral counter-pressure to the side of the head will prevent falling to the affected side. When sitting, the patient should hold his head up and look at the nurse, not downwards. When the patient can do this, he should use this position, i.e. sitting without leaning back, to place his sound foot on the floor, then the affected foot, and then stand up. If help is needed with the affected foot, the nurse should push the leg downwards from above the knee. If, when the affected foot is on the floor, it tends to pull up again, the nurse can, at first, place her foot lightly upon it. When the patient is standing up, the nurse can help him by placing her hand, i.e. the one that is by the patient's sound side, on his back and pushing the lumbar spine forward, so that the hips straighten and enable him to stand upright. At first, he may be allowed to lean against the bed with his thighs.

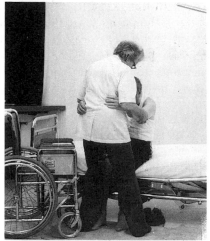

Fig. 6.5a   Patient sitting. Before standing up, patient's affected arm is held round therapist's waist.

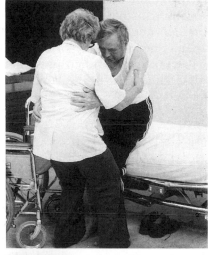

Fig. 6.5b   Patient stands up, moving trunk forward at hips.

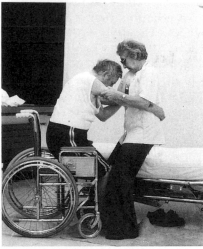

Fig. 6.5c   Patient standing up from, or sitting down into, wheelchair.

If he can stand for a moment without leaning against the bed, the nurse can turn him towards his wheelchair, starting with the upper part of his body and supporting him well under his shoulder and on his back on the sound side. The wheelchair should be placed so that only a quarter-turn is necessary. On sitting down, the upper half of the patient's body should be well forward until he is actually sitting.

Getting up from the chair. The nurse will stand in front of the patient, taking both his hands forward, as for getting up from sitting on the bed. The knees should be together in mid-line and the feet parallel at right angles to the knees. The affected foot should not be in front of the sound one, or at least not far in front of it, as otherwise he will not take weight on it. Should the patient try to raise his affected foot from the floor, the nurse could place her own foot lightly upon it. She should give some pressure on the knee of the affected leg in order to give him the sensation of weightbearing before he stands up, using her hand which is by his sound side. She will then take that hand away from his knee and with it support his back on his lumbar spine and bring his trunk forward. The patient's head should not be bent downward and he should look at the nurse. She will then press her knees against the patient's knees and help him to rise in the same way as she has helped him to rise from the bed (Fig. 6.5c).

Caring for the patient when in the wheelchair

When in a wheelchair, and particularly during the first flaccid stage, the patient will tend to fall towards the affected side. The shouldergirdle and trunk on the affected side falls or pulls downwards and backwards. The head also pulls sideways towards the affected side. If this is not corrected, the patient will later compensate for this tendency by sitting with his whole weight placed on the sound side, always holding tightly to the chair and looking only towards the sound side. This is very unfavourable for rehabilitation of the affected side and for weightbearing and balance and should be corrected early on in sitting.

The chair should have an arm rest wide enough to accommodate and support the arm without letting it slip inward or outward. The arm rest should be long enough to enable the arm to be brought forward as far as possible, allowing the elbow to be extended and preventing retraction of the shoulder. The hand, with the fingers extended in the normal position, can be placed on a circular and rather flat foam rubber support which has been glued to the arm rest (Fig. 6.6a). The arm rest prevents associated flexion and retraction of the arm when the patient wheels the chair himself. A pillow or sandbag should lightly support the affected shoulder to prevent its downward pull. A pillow placed behind the affected shoulder should bring it forward. The patient's trunk should be supported in such a

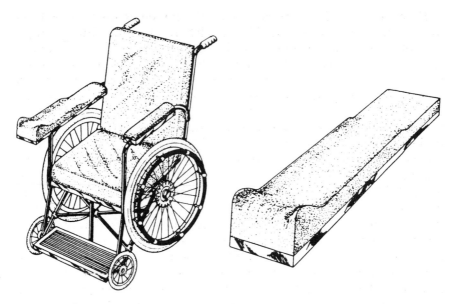

Fig. 6.6a   Drawing of wheelchair and armrest.

way that he cannot lean back; this should be done by means of a board. Care should be taken to see that the affected leg is not abducted. A small sandbag placed against the outside of the thigh will prevent this quite easily.

A still better way than using an arm rest is for the patient to have a removable board in front of him. This allows him to have both arms forward, and he can see his affected arm and hand as well as doing bilateral arm exercises. As he gets used to this position in the wheelchair, he will be well prepared to do the same when sitting at a table. He is taught to hold on to the far edge of the board with his affected hand, a position which brings his shoulder well forward and extends the elbow (Figs. 6.6b, c, d).

Special Points for Attention

In order to help the patient to integrate his affected side into his body image, especially arm and hand, the nurse should pay special attention to the following points:

1.   The patient should sit a great deal with clasped hands and much raising of the arms above his head. He should not 'nurse' the affected hand with the sound one.
2.   He should look towards the affected side.
3.   Visitors and other patients to whom he may be talking, should sit or stand by him on the affected side.

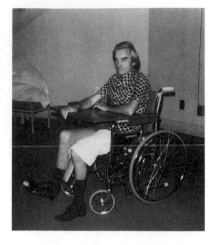

Fig. 6.6b Wheelchair with board in front.
Note: *Patient holding on to board with affected hand.*

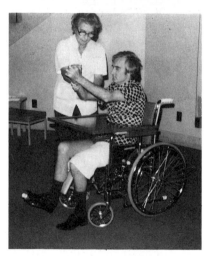

Fig. 6.6c Patient practising bilateral arm movements with clasped hands.

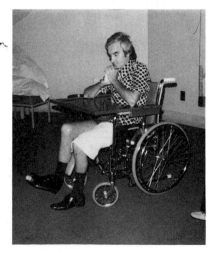

Fig. 6.6d Patient moving clasped hands to mouth.

4. The patient should sit at a table frequently, instead of in a chair without a table in front.
5. He should have both arms on the table, with clasped hands, or, when eating or doing something with his sound hand, the affected arm should lie extended on the table. Also he can be made to hold on to a small upright stick which is fixed on to the table.
6. If help is needed with walking, the nurse should give this on the affected side and never on the sound side.

Physiotherapy in the First (Mainly Flaccid) Stage

Turning over from supine to side-lying

One of the first activities the physiotherapist should work for in treatment is that of turning over to either side. Lying supine is a position which produces maximal extensor spasticity, that is to say retraction of the arm at the shoulder and extensor spasticity of the leg. The patient should not, therefore, always remain in the supine position, but should soon learn to use his trunk, i.e. his shouldergirdle and pelvis, to turn over and lie on his side for some part of the day. If he rolls over and lies on the sound side, with the affected arm uppermost, the shoulder and arm should be moved well forward, the elbow should be extended, and the affected leg lie in a natural position of semi-flexion. If he rolls over and lies on the affected side, the shoulder of that side should, again, be placed well forward, with the elbow extended and in supination. This position helps to prevent shoulder retraction and the development of flexor spasticity with pronation of the affected arm. Positioning in supine has been described in the previous section on nursing care (p. 76).

Rolling over can best be initiated with shouldergirdle and arm movements. The patient, in supine, clasps his hands, the thumb of the affected hand being above that of the sound one to obtain maximal abduction. Clasping his hands together will give him an awareness of equality of both hands, and also some supination of the affected hand. The spreading of the fingers at the metacarpo-phalangeal joints facilitates extension of wrist and fingers and acts against flexor spasticity.

Before rolling over, the patient must practise lifting his clasped hands above his head and down again, with fully extended elbows. The therapist must take care that the palms of both hands have an equal degree of supination (Fig. 6.7a). Then, with his arms extended horizontally forward, he should practise bending his elbows and placing his clasped hands on his chest (Fig. 6.7b). The elbow of the affected arm should be well forward to allow for extension of the wrist. He then moves his arms up again and forward. From this position he

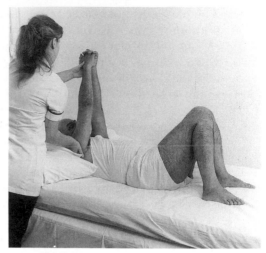

Fig. 6.7a Patient clasps hands. He then raises arms. Note: Shouldergirdle is moved forward and upwards.

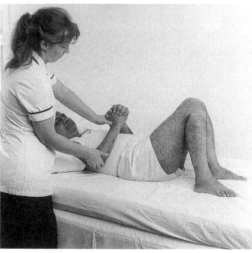

Fig. 6.7b Patient's arms are then moved, with clasped hands to chest.

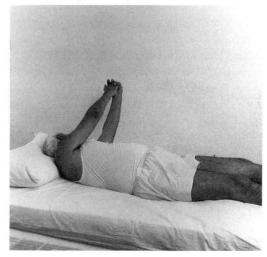

Fig. 6.7c With clasped hands, patient turns towards sound side keeping shoulder well forward.

brings both arms, with clasped hands, over first to one side and then to the other (Fig. 6.7c). He is then helped, if necessary, to move his pelvis and leg over to side-lying. When lying on the affected side, his shoulder should be placed as far forward as possible to counteract retraction of the scapula. The arm is now in external rotation, the forearm supinated and the elbow extended (Fig. 6.8a). This is a 'reflex inhibiting pattern', counteracting flexor spasticity and pronation, and is useful for practising isolated flexion of the elbow, without shoulder retraction, to bring the hand to the mouth, alternating with extension (Fig. 6.8b). The patient can feel his hand touching his mouth, which he enjoys and often sucks his fingers and smiles. It seems that he recognizes and accepts his hand through his mouth more readily than when just looking at his hand. Hand and mouth are closely related in normal child development. The baby learns first about his hand through his mouth, and this seems to be the case also with the hemiplegic patient.

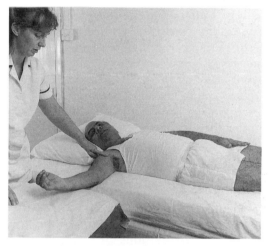

Fig. 6.8a External rotation of the arm in horizontal abduction.
Note; *Shoulder placed forward.*

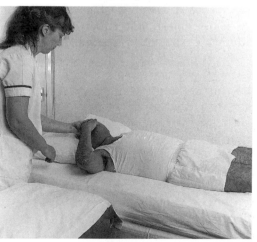

Fig. 6.8b Alternating flexion and extension of elbow and supination of forearm. Hand to face.

Preparing the patient for sitting up and standing

The following treatment sequences should prepare the patient for sitting up from supine through side-lying and from there to standing up. Although, in describing various ways of treatment, a rather artificial division has to be made between working for control of the pelvis and leg and for the shouldergirdle and arm, the therapist must keep in mind at all times that the whole of the affected side is being treated, even if special emphasis is placed on control of leg or arm. Working for control of the arm means working on the shouldergirdle with all its muscular connections to the head, spine and pelvis, i.e. on the trunk. Working for control of the leg means working with the pelvis, with its connections to the spine and shouldergirdle, i.e. again on the trunk. Movements of the arm should start at the shoulder-girdle, and movements of the leg should start at the pelvis. Spasticity of the leg affects the arm and that of the arm affects the leg.

Working for control of the leg. Unfortunately, patients are often made to walk without first having any control of the leg in supine or sitting. Many patients are taught to move and lift the affected leg with the sound one. This is unnecessary in most cases and not only deprives the affected leg of activity during the day, but produces, and increases, extensor and adductor spasticity with supination of the ankle. Furthermore, exercises given in treatment to obtain active flexion will not have a carry-over into daily function, as the patient will find it easier to lift the affected leg passively with the sound one. He gets used to doing it and continues to do it, even if, later on, he is capable of lifting his affected leg actively.

Flexion and lifting of the leg. During all treatment for control of the leg, great care should be taken to avoid associated flexion of the arm and retraction of the shoulder. This can be done in supine by the patient holding his hands clasped and lifted above his head. Should this be too difficult for him, i.e. if there is shoulder pain, his arm can be placed extended by his side. If flexion should occur due to the patient making an effort, the therapist should lift his arm, inhibit flexor spasticity and then place it down again in extension.

Flexion of the leg at hip and knee — and, even more so, flexion of the knee with the hip extended, which is necessary for walking without circumduction — is difficult, because any activity results in excessive and uncontrolled extension of the leg. When trying to bend and lift the leg, co-contraction occurs, i.e. simultaneous contraction of the extensors and the flexor groups of muscles. The contraction of the extensors may be so strong that the patient extends his leg before he tries to bend it. The leg is then heavy, drops down again and resists flexion afterwards. In treatment, therefore, it is important first to obtain controlled extension without extensor spasticity, so that unresisted flexion is possible and easy for the patient. This is done in the following way:

> The therapist bends the patient's leg, but avoids it falling into abduction, which is part of the total abnormal flexor pattern. The foot is held in dorsiflexion and pronation. The therapist waits until all resistance has subsided and then slowly, and in stages, extends the leg, asking the patient not to let the leg fall or push against her hand. When at any stage of this movement she feels the full weight of the leg or even the slightest push against her hand, she stops the movement and asks the patient to bend the leg a little until he holds and controls it again.

He thus learns to reverse the movement, using flexion against extension, and actively inhibits extensor spasticity. Gradually, he should learn to control the full range of extension and be able to reverse the movement at any stage. The only support given is at the sole of the foot; the ball of the toes should not be touched as this would increase extensor spasticity (Figs. 6.9a, b). On the way towards full extension, the foot should be kept near the support, so that the movement resembles that needed in walking. Straight leg raising should not be practised, as it has no functional significance and increases extensor spasticity at knee and ankle. When the patient can control his leg in some degree of flexion, with his heel firmly on the support, active dorsiflexion of the ankle can be practised. The therapist dorsiflexes the foot by giving some pressure backwards and downwards against the ankle, while, with her other hand, she lifts the front of the foot, with the toes dorsiflexed. The lateral border of the foot should be raised more than the medial one to maintain pronation (Fig. 6.9c). When resistance has subsided in full dorsiflexion, the patient should be asked to hold the foot up, and not to press his toes down when the therapist lowers it. If he can control this, he will be able to assist the next movement of dorsiflexion. Dorsiflexion with eversion of the ankle can be reinforced by dorsiflexion of the toes. It can be done by sensory stimulation with quick stroking movements along the plantar aspect of the toes, excluding the big toe (Fig. 6.9d).

Extension in preparation for weightbearing. Extension without extensor spasticity in preparation for weightbearing should now be practised. The therapist places the patient's dorsiflexed and pronated foot against herself, holds it in this position and asks the patient to perform small isolated movements of alternate flexion and extension of the knee. With her hand under his knee, she may give some resistance to extension when he moves the back of his knee down against her hand. This produces selective quadriceps contractions alternating with slight flexion, and will prepare for weightbearing without hyperextension (back-kneeing) later on (Fig. 6.10).

When the patient can control his leg during the extensor phase, the

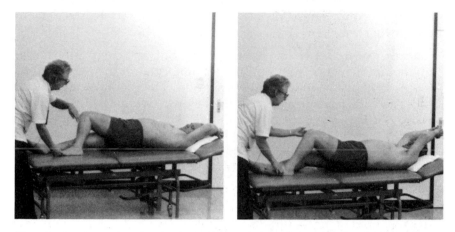

Fig 6.9a, b   In supine, leg is placed in varying degrees of flexion with adduction.
Note: *Patient should control intermediate position and not push into extension.*

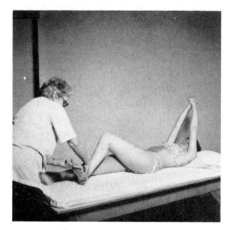
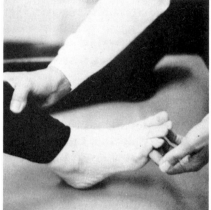

Fig. 6.9c   Working with active dorsi-flexion of ankle and toes.
Note: *Lateral border of foot raised and backward pressure applied to ankle.*

Fig. 6.9d   Stroking plantar aspect of toes to obtain dorsiflextion.

therapist, supporting his foot as above, helps him to bend the leg and move the foot down over the side of the bed or plinth so that he extends his hip with the knee in flexion. From there, he should lift his leg up again and place his foot on the support. If the patient is able to do this by himself, there will be no need for him to move the affected leg with the sound one for sitting up.

Preparing for walking without circumduction

The following ways of treatment are useful in preparation for walking without circumduction.

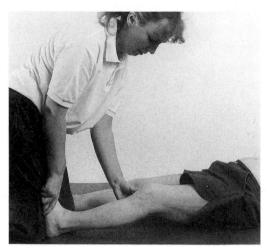

Fig. 6.10   Extension of knee
with dorsiflexed foot.

With the patient's leg down over the side of the bed or plinth, and his hip extended, the therapist supports his foot in dorsiflexion and helps him to bend his knee as far as possible without bending his hip. This is alternated with extension, but care should be taken not to extend the knee further than can be done without extensor spasm. If extensor spasticity occurs, the patient cannot bend the knee again. The range of extension should gradually be increased, but only as long as the patient can reverse the movement. It often helps to have the sole of the foot sliding along the ground when bending the knee, but dorsiflexion and pronation should be maintained (Figs. 6.11a, b).

With the patient's foot on the bed or plinth and his knee in flexion, the sound leg extended, he is asked and helped to adduct the leg and to rotate his pelvis forward on the affected side. Adduction may be resisted when the leg is flexed, and the therapist may have to elongate the whole of the affected side, i.e. the side-flexors of the trunk and the abductors of the leg. With the pelvis rotated well forward and lifted on the affected side, hip extension with a flexed knee is obtained, a pattern which is much needed for walking. The foot is then in a

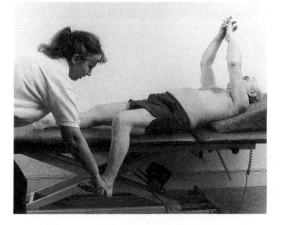

Fig. 6.11a   Flexion of knee
while hip extends when putting foot down.

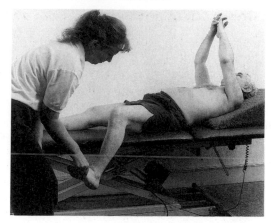

Fig. 6.11b With hips now extended, knee resists flexion.

position of dorsiflexion and pronation and the patient can use it to help to push the pelvis forward towards the sound side and extend his hip (Fig. 6.12a). Then, with the pelvis rotated forward, the leg can be moved across the sound one, the foot touching a wall with its medial border (Fig. 6.12b). Isolated flexion and extension of the knee may then be practised, the foot moving up and down the wall. Often, the patient is then able to dorsiflex the toes, especially if the therapist has mobilized them against the usual plantiflexion.

Fig. 6.12a Extension of hip with flexed knee. Patient pushes with foot and rotates pelvis forward.

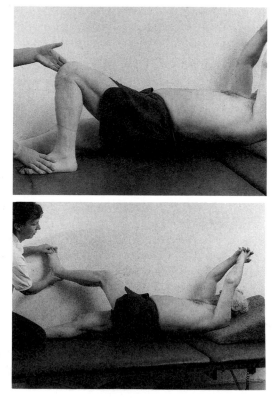

Fig. 6.12b Moving leg up and down with foot placed against a wall, using selective flexion and extension of knee.

Control of adduction and abduction at the hip in supine

Many patients lack this control of adduction and abduction, yet are still expected to walk. To obtain control, the patient lies with both legs flexed and his feet flat on the support. The affected foot should remain parallel with and near to the sound one but, to begin with, it may have to be prevented from slipping forward into extension. The patient should hold and keep the sound knee steady in mid-position, i.e. he should not move it when asked to perform small movements of adduction and abduction, alternately, with the affected leg. He should learn to arrest and hold the process of these movements exactly where and when he is asked to do so. At first, he may overshoot the desired position, or be unable to reverse the movement, especially if the leg tends to fall outwards into abduction. When he has gained control of these movements, he is asked to keep the affected leg steady in mid-line and to adduct and abduct the sound leg. The independent holding of the affected leg when moving the sound one is very important for later walking, as otherwise there will be no control and fixation of the affected leg at the hip when making a step with the sound leg.

The same manoeuvre can be practised later on with the pelvis raised off the support. If this is possible and done well, the patient can next lift one foot off the bed or plinth and support himself only on the other, but when he lifts the sound leg, his pelvis should be level and not allowed to drop on the affected side.

Sitting up from supine and side-lying

Sitting up from supine and side-lying has been described under *Positioning and Moving for Nurses and Therapists, see* pp. 80–83.

Trunk balance in sitting

When sitting, the patient tends to fall to the affected side. He is afraid of doing so and in consequence does not put weight on to the affected hip. Flexor spasticity pulls his head and neck laterally towards the affected side, together with the side-flexors of his trunk. This flexor pattern reinforces flexion of his arm and pressure downwards of the shouldergirdle, and prevents extension and arm support on the affected side. In sitting and standing, balancing without arm support when weightbearing on one side makes the normal person move his head laterally towards the opposite side. It is surprising that the sound side of a hemiplegic patient is unable to counteract the pull or fall to the affected side. It may be due to the pull of spastic muscles towards the affected side, and also to sensory loss, depriving the sound side of information about what happens on the affected side. Whatever the reason, the patient will not feel safe enough to use the affected side for weightbearing and balance unless he gets trunk control with righting of his head towards the sound side. For this he needs elongation of the side-flexors of trunk and neck, and raising of his shouldergirdle on the affected side. This should be combined, as soon as possible, with support on his forearm and, later, on his extended arm.

In treatment, the patient sits on the bed or plinth with the therapist on his affected side. She raises his shouldergirdle supporting it from under the axilla, holding his arm abducted in lateral rotation,* extended at the elbow, the hand extended at the wrist with the fingers, if possible, also extended. The patient should not support himself with his sound hand, but rather place that hand on his knee, or better still, lift it up. He then should lean towards the therapist, and straighten himself up again to the mid-position. He should start this by side-flexing his head laterally to the sound side and not just turn his head. When moving to the affected side, he should not lean backwards. The shouldergirdle should be kept raised by the therapist. Next, the patient's hand is placed on the support some distance away from the body, the therapist holding the hand firmly down while lifting his shouldergirdle up with her other hand. The patient is then asked to move his trunk towards the therapist so that he takes full weight on the affected hip (Fig. 6.13a). The patient is then helped to take weight on his forearm, his hands clasped, or his hand being held flat down on the support either with his sound hand or by the therapist. If he feels very insecure and tends to collaspe on his arm, his shouldergirdle can be kept raised by the therapist or, alternatively, if

* Lateral rotation equals external or outward rotation, medial rotation equals internal or inward rotation.

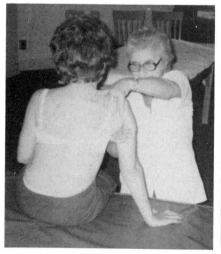

Fig. 6.13a Weight transfer to affected side with support on extended arm.

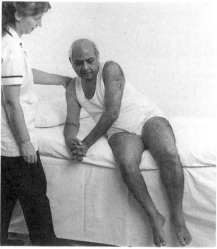

Fig. 6.13b Weightbearing in sitting on affected side with support on forearm.

possible, she should just keep his head laterally flexed towards the sound side to stop his pulling down or falling to the affected side (Fig. 6.13b). It is always difficult for the patient to lean forward at his hips when sitting without being afraid of falling forward. It is important to practise this for balance as well as for standing up. The therapist stands in front of the patient, fixing his affected extended arm against her waist with her elbow, and letting him hold on to her with his sound one. He is then asked, and helped, to lean well forward at the hips (Fig. 6.14a). Care should be taken to see that he extends his back

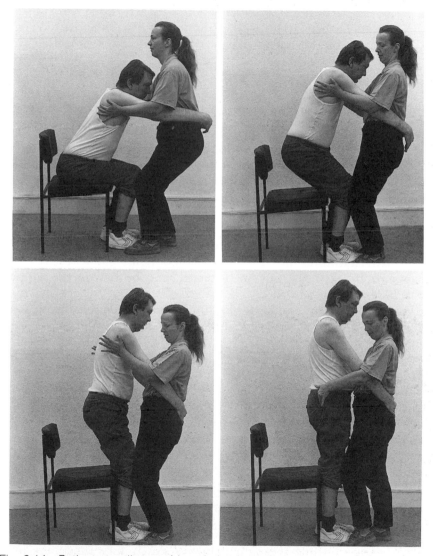

Fig. 6.14   Patient standing up (description in text).
Note: *(a) Patient takes weight first on flexed hips and knees. (b) He is then helped by the therapist to extend hips and bring them forward. (c) Therapist's knee is pushing against patient's knee. (d) Patient stands up.*

and does not bend his head and look down. From this position, he is then helped to stand up, as has been described before under *Positioning and Moving the Patient* p. 84 (Figs. 6.14b, c, d).

Working for extended arm support in sitting

The practice of support and weightbearing on extended arm is important for two reasons:

1. Extension, with outward rotation, abduction and supination counteracts flexor spasticity which is associated with inward rotation, pronation and retraction of the shoulder. Weight-bearing on the extended arm activates the extensor muscles in a much needed functional pattern.
2. Weightbearing on the extended arm is part of the process of gaining balance and makes the patient feel sufficiently safe to bear weight on the affected side without fear of falling over.

Weightbearing can be practised in the following ways. The patient's hand is placed on the support some distance away from his body. His shouldergirdle is lifted and supported under the axilla by the therapist. He moves his trunk well over his supporting arm, transferring most of his weight on to the affected hip. This elongates the side-flexors of the trunk on that side and brings the shoulder up and vertically over his hand. He may not then need support under the axilla and the therapist can support his elbow in full extension. To avoid internal rotation, his hand should point sideways, or even diagonally backwards, but not forward, and be flat on the support with his fingers extended.

When the patient can keep his elbow extended without help, some downward pressure can be given to his shoulder to increase extensor activity and stability. He is then asked to perform small selective movements of his elbow, i.e. slight flexion alternating with full extension (Figs. 6.15a, b).

If flexor spasticity is very strong and the patient cannot keep his arm extended by his side, it can be inhibited by moving his arm backward in extension and full external rotation. The therapist is now behind the patient. The patient's hand is supported with his wrist extended. In order to keep the shoulders level and to prevent the sound shoulder from moving forward, which would reduce the effect of the manoeuvre, the sound hand can be held in the same way at the same time, so that both arms are extended backwards. The therapist can also ask the patient to place his sound hand backwards on the support. When moving both arms backwards, she can also lift them off the support while the patient moves slowly forward at the hips. This produces good extension of the spine and also of the arms. Gentle alternating push and pull will stimulate active extension (Figs. 6.16a, b).

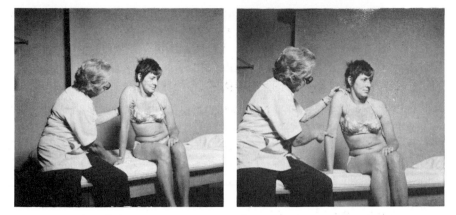

Figs. 6.15a, b   Sitting with support on affected arm, shoulder well raised, the patient performs small isolated movements of elbow. Also she moves her trunk forward, backward and sideways.

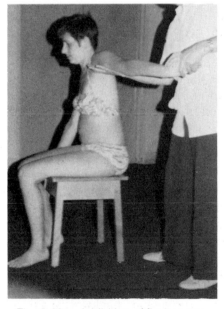

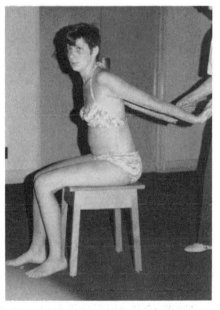

Fig. 6.16a   Inhibition of flexor spasticity of affected arm.
Note: *Shouldergirdle is raised to counteract pressure down. The patient moves trunk and shouldergirdle while the therapist inhibits flexor spasticity.*

Fig. 6.16b   Gentle push-pull stimulates active extension of the arm.

This can be followed either by placing his affected hand sideways on the support, as described above, or by lifting his extended arm sideways up, continuing to give a gentle pull and push. The patient

ep his arm extended and, to begin with, may need some
the elbow.

...ol of the arm at the shoulder

It is easier for the patient to get control of his shouldergirdle and arm in supine than in sitting, because when the hips are flexed, the tendency to flexor spasticity is increased.

During all work for extension and lifting of the arm, the patient's leg should be in some flexion, with the foot pronated and the sole on the support. The leg should be adducted with the pelvis rotated forward towards the sound side to prevent the flexed leg from abducting and the pelvis from pulling backwards. It is essential to maintain flexion of the leg in order to avoid the occurrence of extensor spasticity, through associated reactions, especially when the patient makes an effort to lift his arm or to hold it up.

Mobilizing the shouldergirdle

Mobility of the scapula is important not only to obtain movements of the arm at the shoulder, but also to prevent shoulder pain. In all cases, even in those where the arm is flaccid, we find a combination of flexor spasticity of the side-flexors of the trunk, depression and retraction of the shoulder and fixation of the scapula. Spasticity of the rhomboids, trapezius and latissimus prevents the inferior angle of the scapula from turning outwards and upwards when the arm is raised. If the scapula cannot move freely, passive lifting of the arm above the horizontal, especially if done with internal rotation, pushes the humerus against the acromion, with the supraspinatus and the capsule pressed against it, which is painful.

Mobilizing the shouldergirdle can be done best in supine, but can also be done in side-lying on the sound side. The aim is to make the painless elevation of the arm possible. The patient's arm is supported by the therapist with his elbow extended and in external rotation. She uses both hands to move his shouldergirdle upwards, forward and downward, but avoids moving it backwards as this reinforces retraction of the scapula. The patient's head should be laterally flexed towards the sound side. If shoulder retraction is very strong, the procedure can be done in side-lying on the sound side. The shouldergirdle is then more easily brought forward (Figs. 6.17a, b, c, d).

Another way of mobilizing the shouldergirdle is to extend the patient's arm above his head, with his hand held firmly in this position, the arm in external rotation. He is then asked to turn over into side- and prone-lying, i.e. he moves his body against the arm. When on his side, he may need help to move his shoulder well forward. Moving the trunk against the limb is reducing spasticity

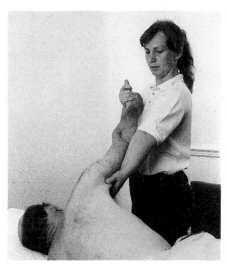

Fig. 6.17a Patient in sidelying: mobilizing shouldergirdle.
Note: Shoulder and scapula are moved upwards and forwards.

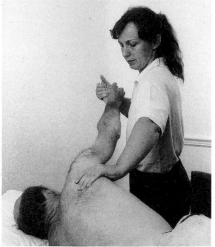

Fig. 6.17b This is done with the arm in external rotation.

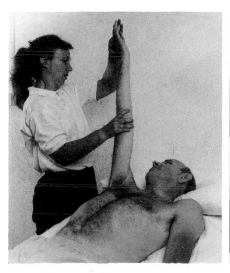

Fig. 6.17c Patient in supine: mobilizing shouldergirdle forward and upwards with arm in extension and supination.

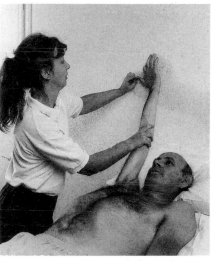

Fig. 6.17d This is followed by elevating arm and placing palm of hand against wall.
Note: Abduction of thumb.

more effectively than pulling the arm against the trunk. The whole of the affected side becomes maximally elongated. In this way, using rotation, the patient counteracts his flexor spasticity actively (Figs. 6.18a, b, c, d).

When resistance to moving the shouldergirdle is no longer present, the therapist gradually raises the extended arm in supine, using some

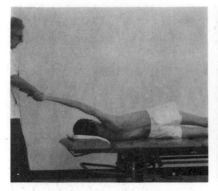

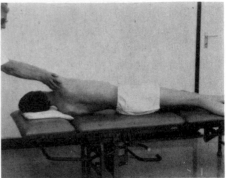

Fig. 6.18a Shoulder retraction makes patient start movement from the pelvis.

Fig. 6.18b Therapist now helps patient by mobilizing shouldergirdle and trunk and bringing it forward.

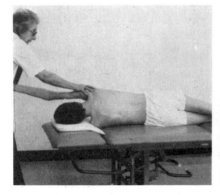

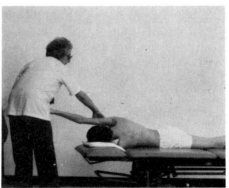

Fig. 6.18c Note: *Elongation of the whole of the affected side as the turning movement goes on.*

Fig. 6.18d Movement almost completed.
Note: *Elongation of affected side maintained throughout.*

traction and keeping the shoulder well forward. At the first indication of shoulder pain, the upward movement must be stopped and the arm slightly lowered again. Shoulder pain occurs when the patient pulls the scapula back and downwards. The arm is then slowly moved up again until full elevation has been obtained without pain. The whole pattern of the flexor synergy has to be counteracted by elongating the side of the trunk, by movement of the shoulder forward and upward, by external rotation of the arm, and by keeping the elbow and wrist extended, with the fingers also extended, if possible (Fig. 6.19a).

As soon as there is no resistance to the arm in full elevation, the patient is encouraged to extend his elbow actively, while his hand is still suppported in extension. He is asked to push upwards against the

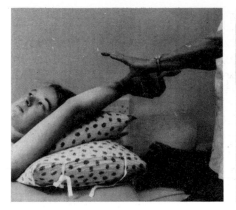
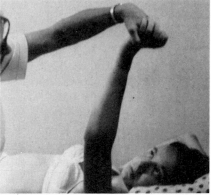

Fig. 6.19a   Elevation of arm. This is
done with extension and external
rotation.

Fig. 6.19b   The patient pushes in-
termittently upwards against the
therapist's hand with alternating
slight and isolated flexion and extension of elbow.

therapist's hand. Alternate small movements of flexion and extension
at the elbow are practised to obtain selective movements of the elbow
(Fig. 6.19b). When the patient is able to do this, the therapist releases
his hand and the patient tries to keep the arm up unaided and then to
move it a little at the shoulder without letting it fall sideways or
forward and down. All forward movements, i.e. into flexion, are more
difficult for him to control than adduction and abduction of the
shoulder. He should only move as far as he can control and reverse the
movements, i.e. lift his arm up again. Later, he should learn to arrest
the downward movement of his arm at any intermediate stage and
from these points lift the arm up again. In the end, he should be able
to lift his arm up from his side with his elbow still extended. At first,
the therapist may have to keep the shoulder forward to stabilize the
shouldergirdle.

STAGE OF SPASTICITY

The gradual development of spasticity occurs during the first stage,
i.e. the mainly flaccid stage. The treatment during these two stages,
therefore, overlaps, and some treatment done in supine, for instance,
will have to be continued, but progressed towards sitting and
standing.

When spasticity has developed, the process of spontaneous recovery
is often arrested. It is at this stage that most patients with residual
hemiplegia come for out-patient treatment.

Spasticity usually develops slowly with a predilection for the flexor
muscles of the upper, and the extensor muscles of the lower limbs. It
usually increases with the patient's activities and use of effort

throughout the first 18 months. Some patients, however, develop strong spasticity quite early, that is to say within a few days. As spasticity develops, there is increasing resistance to certain passive movements. The muscle groups most affected are the depressors of shouldergirdle and arm, the fixators and retractors of the scapula, the side-flexors of the trunk, the adductors and internal rotators of the arm, the flexors and pronators of the elbow and wrist, and the flexors and adductors of the fingers. In the leg, spasticity is most pronounced in the extensors of the hip, knee and ankle, and in the supinators of the feet. The toes may be in dorsiflexion, while the ankle is plantiflexed, but if the ankle is passively dorsiflexed, the toes plantiflex and give resistance to dorsiflexion. This 'shifting' of spasticity can also be observed in the hand. Some patients show strong flexor spasticity of the elbow and wrist, the fingers being more or less extended. When extending the elbow and wrist passively, however, the fingers flex and resist extension.

The testing of individual muscles or muscle groups for spasticity by assessing resistance to passive stretch without taking into account the position of the patient's head and trunk or of his proximal joints will give different and misleading results. For instance, in a patient with flexor spasticity of the arm, resistance to extension of the elbow is strong when the arm is at the side of the patient's body. If, however, the arm is raised and moved forward to the horizontal at the shoulder, there will be less resistance to passive flexion. If the patient sits, and leans forward and downwards with his trunk, the arm may extend stiffly at the elbow and resist flexion. If the arm is elevated passively, the elbow extends and flexion is resisted. This shows the difficulty which occurs when the therapist tries to place the patient's hand to his face or to the crown of his head with the arm lifted up at the shoulder. These few examples show the variability of the degree and distribution of spasticity when testing isolated muscles. Also, such testing does not give any information about functional use. Therefore, it is better and more reliable to test for spasticity with movements which the patient cannot perform. For instance, elevation of the arm with flexed elbow, supination of the forearm with extended elbow and extended wrist and fingers, abduction of the arm with extended elbow, wrist and fingers, etc. This way of testing gives the necessary information, not only of resistance to functional patterns, but also for treatment which aims at inhibition of the spastic patterns which interfere with them.

Whereas spasticity is transient during the flaccid stage, more constant hypertonicity is found during the second stage. The arm and leg take up a permanent and fairly typical posture, the arm and hand in flexion, internal rotation and pronation, the leg in extension with the foot plantified and supinated.

If spasticity is moderate, the patient is able to bend his leg, but only with abduction and in a total pattern of flexion. In trying to overcome the resistance of spastic extensor muscles, he has to use excessive effort. When he extends his leg, he has no control over the various stages of extension or flexion and he is unable to arrest the movement at any intermediate stage. In order to bend his knee, he has first to lift his leg with the knee extended until there is enough hip flexion to make flexion of the knee possible. Straight leg raising, however, has no functional use for walking, and should not, therefore, be practised. The patient cannot keep his foot on the support when bending his leg and he should learn to do this from the beginning. The lack of control over extension has a detrimental effect on walking, as the patient will drop his leg, or push it down when making a step. The leg, and especially the ankle, is then stiff, the ball of the foot touches the ground first and presses against it. Dorsiflexion of the ankle is lacking, making weight transfer over the standing leg difficult or impossible, resulting in hyperextension of the knee. The leg is then too stiff to allow it to be easily lifted for making the next step. In order to prepare for more normal walking, it is first essential to obtain controlled extension in supine lying, i.e. inhibition of extensor spasticity. Dorsiflexion of the foot at the ankle may be possible with the leg in flexion, provided the ankle is pronated, but it is impossible with the leg extended.

When sitting, the patient carries more weight on the sound hip than on the affected one. The affected arm is flexed, the leg, if flexed at the knee is more widely abducted than the sound one, but if there is strong extensor spasticity, the knee is in some degree of extension and the leg adducted. There is side flexion of the trunk, and the shoulder on the affected side is held lower than that on the sound side. When standing up, the affected foot is in front of the sound one and all the weight is taken on the sound leg, while the patient pushes himself up with the sound arm. The patient can usually stand at this stage, but nearly all his weight is supported on the sound leg. He cannot stand on a small base and he will learn to walk in an abnormal manner. He may hold the affected leg in extension and external rotation, swinging it forward by lifting and pulling the pelvis up on the affected side. He circumducts the extended leg and places the foot down in pronation to get the heel to the ground. In a few cases where the leg is less stiff, the patient will lean the trunk backwards and push the pelvis and leg forward to make a step. In other cases, the patient may bend the hip and knee to some extent when making a step forward using less circumduction but, if the foot is plantiflexed and supinated, he may be unable to put his heel to the ground and his ankle tends to turn over. If spasticity is slight, the heel is placed down after the toes have touched the ground. The spastic resistance of the calf muscles makes full dorsiflexion in weightbearing and weight transfer forward of the hip impossible. The patient, therefore, bends his trunk forward at the hip in order to transfer his weight over the standing leg. This results in hyperextension of his knee.

The effort used in lifting his stiffly extended leg in walking increases the flexor spasticity of his arm. This is due to associated reactions which are strong at this stage of spasticity. The patient uses his affected leg as a rigid 'prop' (co-contraction) to take his weight in standing and walking, for without extensor spasticity and co-contraction his leg will collapse. In a few cases, there may be elements of flexor spasticity, making it difficult for the patient to put his foot down to the ground after having moved it forward for a step. The constant use of these abnormal motor patterns will increase flexor spasticity of the arm and extensor spasticity in the leg.

Movements of the arm are restricted to one pattern. When trying to raise the arm, the patient uses the whole of the affected side and often just lifts his shouldergirdle with some abduction of the arm at the shoulder. The elbow remains flexed, or it may flex even more than it did before he tried to lift the arm. He cannot lift the extended arm forward or sideways up, and is unable to supinate his forearm or move his wrist and fingers. A few patients carry the arm flexed and supinated, with strong retraction at the shoulder. Independent movements at the elbow are impossible.

Subluxation of the arm at the shoulder becomes a problem in many patients when they are upright, i.e. sitting, standing and walking, especially so in those who will show any degree of flaccidity of, for instance, the deltoid and supraspinatus. However, there is always some evidence of spasticity in the predominantly flaccid arm. There is a tendency to flexion of wrist and fingers, and spasticity of the lateral flexors of the neck and those around the scapula. The shouldergirdle is retracted and resists being moved forward, the inferior angle of the scapula is fixed and does not move laterally and upwards when the arm is lifted. The acromion, therefore, does not turn upward to maintain the head of the humerus in the glenoid fossa. It is not only gravity which pulls the arm down and out of the glenohumeral joint, but also spasticity of the depressors of the humerus, i.e. of the subscapularis, infraspinatus and teres minor. The adductors and medial rotators, i.e. pectoralis major and latissimus dorsi as well as the side-flexors of the trunk, reinforce the pattern of flexion and depression of the shouldergirdle (Davies, 1985).

Subluxation does not produce shoulder pain on elevating the patient's arm passively as long as the scapula is mobile and there is no resistance to moving it forward and upward. However, if rotation and abduction of the scapula is prevented by spasticity and fixation by the rhomboids and trapezius, the glenoid fossa remains turned down-wards instead of upwards, and passive lifting of the arm above the horizontal plane produces pain as the capsule and supraspinatus are pressed against the acromion. This is especially so if the arm is internally rotated and the shoulder retracted. Basmajian (1962) has described the causes for subluxation and mentioned the importance of rotation of the scapula in great detail. He says:

'At the shoulder joint, we have found that the main muscular activity in resisting downward dislocation occurs in supraspinatus (and to a slight extent in the posterior, horizontal running fibres of the deltoid). The bulk of the deltoid, and the biceps and triceps shows no activity in spite of their vertical direction. Surprisingly, this is true even when heavy weights are suspended from the arm. The function of supraspinatus is apparently associated with a previously undescribed locking mechanism dependent upon the slope of the glenoid fossa. The horizontal pull of the muscle, along with an extreme tightening of the superior part of the capsule when the arm hangs down vertically, prevents downward subluxation of the humeral head.'

The wearing of a sling is supposed to push the humerus upwards mechanically and so prevent subluxation. However, as the arm is in flexion, adducted, pronated and internally rotated in the sling, flexor spasticity, which is the main cause of subluxation, is reinforced. Moreover, inactivity and wasting of those muscles which should counteract flexor spasticity and make raising the arm possible, such as serratus magnus, deltoid, supraspinatus and the extensors of the elbow, cannot be avoided, while the spasticity of the flexor synergy, i.e. pectorals, internal rotators and adductors of the arm and scapula, as well as of the flexors of the forearm, is increased. Oedema of the hand lying flexed in the sling may become an additional problem.

In the early stages, before the patient can use active extension—lifting and holding the arm up against gravity—a temporary support may be given to the shouldergirdle to prevent long-lasting stretch of the superior part of the capsule and supraspinatus. The patient will need this support when he is upright until such time as he can use the supraspinatus and deltoid to hold the humeral head in the glenoid fossa. Such support should consist of a 'cuff' applied to the upper arm and held by a figure-of-eight bandage (Williams et al., 1988). So far, we have used a small and soft foam rubber cushion under the axilla, which abducts the arm slightly, but may tend to displace the head of the humerus laterally (Figs. 6.20a, b, c, d).

Such support of the upper arm keeps it mobile and leaves the elbow free to extend. If it should be necessary to prevent the arm from hanging down, the patient could be made to put his hand into a pocket by his side. However, this is advisable and necessary in only a few flaccid patients, and has the disadvantage of maintaining the fingers in flexion. To obtain extension of wrist and fingers, a foam rubber 'finger-spreader' can be used, which abducts fingers and thumb. Abduction not only facilitates extension of the fingers, but also reduces flexor spasticity throughout the whole arm. The patient finds this comfortable and should also use the 'finger-spreader' when sleeping. It has a better and more dynamic effect than the use of a splint and reduces the possibility of oedema (Fig6.21).

When the patient does not need to use the sound hand for any task, he should sit with his fingers clasped, instead of the usual way of

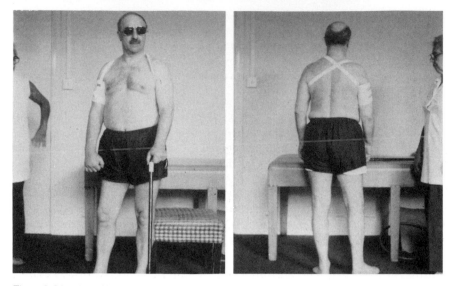

Figs. 6.20a, b   Method of preventing subluxation of the shoulder. 'Cuff' support of arm to raise head of humerus fixed to trunk by figure-of-eight bandage.

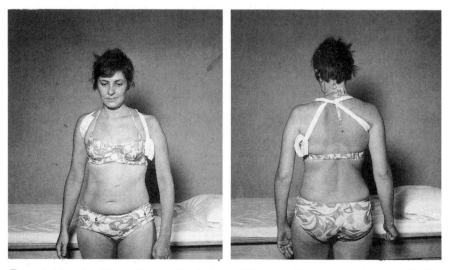

Figs. 6.20c, d   Alternative method. A small foam rubber support placed in the axilla is held in place by the same means.

'nursing' his affected hand with the sound one. Clasping the hands has the same effect as the 'finger-spreader'—it reduces flexor spasticity and gives extension through abduction of fingers and thumb, and has the added advantage of keeping the forearm in supination. The patient then sees both his arms and his hands in front of him and gets the feeling of bilaterality. The affected hand then looks, and perhaps feels, more like the sound one and, therefore, becomes more acceptable as part of his body percept again. If possible, the patient

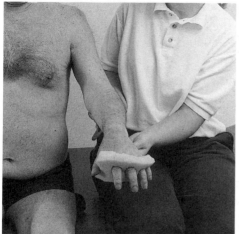

Fig. 6.21 Foam rubber 'finger spreader' to obtain extension and abduction of fingers and thumb. This should be worn in between treatment sessions in support of treatment.

should sit at a table or, if in a wheelchair, with a tray in front of him, so that his upper arm is supported and raised forward.

Treatment at the Second Stage

Treatment at this stage is a progression of that given in the first stage. Though much of the treatment will now be done in sitting and standing, some of the previous activities should be continued. Whereas, in the first stage, extension, external rotation, abduction and elevation of the whole arm, and flexion of the leg at all joints, were the aim, a breaking-up of these total patterns is now needed in order to obtain better adaptation of movements to functional and selective skills.

It is of primary importance for the patient to get up as soon as possible after a stroke, in order to get weight on the affected side in sitting and standing*. In the case of hemiplegic patients, who are already walking badly, especially those with a long-standing condition who cannot walk without a tripod or stick, the therapist has to decide whether it is more important to work for balance in standing and walking, or to work for and improve the use of arm and hand. However, it must be realized, and borne in mind, that no separation of leg or arm activity should be made, even if the emphasis of treatment is placed, temporarily, on one or the other. We always have to remember that lack of balance and difficulty in moving the affected leg in walking will increase flexor spasticity in the arm and hand, and that effort and abnormal walking will prevent any potential use of the affected arm. On the other hand, decrease of spasticity in trunk and arm will decrease the extensor spasticity of the leg and make easier and more normal movements of the leg possible in standing and

* This depends on the doctor's permission.

walking. Whichever function it is decided to emphasize in treatment, therefore, the affected side, i.e. the trunk together with the arm and leg, must always be treated as a whole.

Treatment in sitting and standing up

By now, the patient has control of his trunk and does not tend to fall towards the affected side. However, he does not carry his full weight on the affected hip as he has insufficient balance on that side. At home, he likes to sit in a comfortable easy chair, or in a wheelchair, where he can lean backwards. This does not give him any opportunity to practise the balance reactions he needs. In this position of half-lying, his hip and leg are semi-extended and his knee too stiff to bend, which means that he cannot bring his heel backwards under the chair for standing up. He should, therefore, as soon as possible, learn to sit safely on an ordinary chair at home or, in treatment, on a stool without a back rest. His affected foot should not be in front of the sound one, and equal weight should be on both hips or, preferably, at least in treatment, more weight should be on the affected one. When his leg is well flexed at hip and knee, it tends to abduct more than the sound one—it actually falls outward. Then passive adduction may be resisted and active adduction may be difficult, due to retraction and backward rotation of the pelvis and trunk on that side. For treatment, it is useful to have the patient sitting on the middle chair of three, or have one chair to sit on and another by the affected side, as he is more afraid of transferring weight to the affected side if there is nothing to support him there. It also gives the therapist a chance to practise arm support. He can then learn to shift himself from one chair to another.

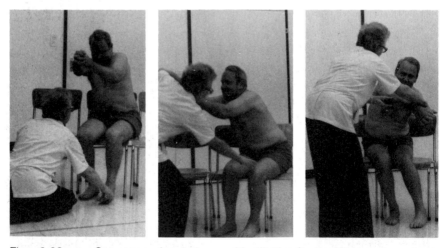

Figs. 6.22a–c Sequence of techniques of facilitation for standing up. Learning to control standing up and shifting pelvis from side to side without use of arms and hands. Rotation of pelvis against shouldergirdle and movement of trunk against pelvis.

Finding the centre of a chair with his hips without looking helps him to gain control of his pelvis. It also makes rotation of his trunk and elongation of the affected side possible, especially when he moves himself towards that side. He should do all this with his trunk and arms moved well forward and his hands clasped. The same procedure can also be done sitting on a low plinth (Figs. 6.22a, b, c).

Control of adduction and abduction in sitting can be practised as done before in supine (p. 97). If the patient finds adduction with a flexed leg difficult, the therapist may feel resistance when she does it passively. She can then help and reduce this resistance by getting forward rotation of the pelvis, with the patient moving both legs towards the sound side, his knees remaining close together. She can also help the patient to lift his leg and cross it over the sound one. Sitting in this position at home sometimes will also be of help. He should sit with his hands clasped around his knee (Figs. 6.23a, b).

The patient usually finds it very difficult to lift his leg and the reason for this becomes clear when the therapist lifts it passively. She will not only feel the whole weight of the leg, but also pressure downwards. When she puts her hand under his foot while it is still on the ground, she will feel pressure of the ball of the foot and of the toes against her hand—a result of extensor spasticity. The patient, therefore, has to overcome this resistance when asked to lift his leg, which to him feels like a heavy weight. The therapist should explain to him that it is not because he is too weak to lift it, but because he pushes his leg down. This can be proved to him by flexing it up passively until there is no resistance in full flexion and then very

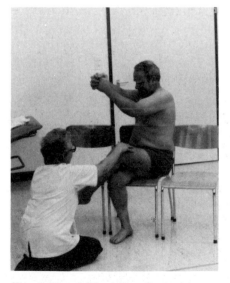

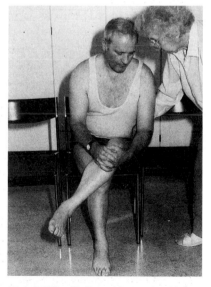

Fig. 6.23a Lifting the affected leg and crossing it over the sound one.

Fig. 6.23b Sitting with crossed legs. Note: The spastic leg over the sound one.

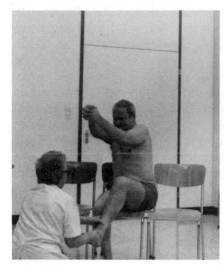 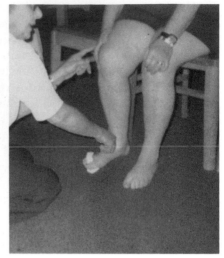

Fig. 6.24 Lowering flexed, affected leg slowly. The patient holds and controls each stage.

Fig. 6.25 Moving dorsiflexed foot backwards prior to standing up.

slowly lowering it, asking him to hold and control it until the foot touches the ground without pressure. He will now be able to lift it up with greater ease, but the therapist must keep her hand lightly under the dorsiflexed foot so that she can keep a check on any degree of downward pressure which will interfere with his lifting the leg actively (Fig. 6.24).

Bending the knee and moving the foot backward under the chair with the heel remaining on the ground is another difficulty to overcome, but is essential in preparation for standing up with the weight on the affected leg. This movement pattern will also benefit the patient's walking when he needs independent flexion of his knee before making a step forward (Fig. 6.25).

Treatment for standing up and standing

When standing up, the patient immediately pulls the sound foot backward under the chair, but the knee of the affected leg cannot bend sufficiently to do this. The affected foot is always in front of the sound one and the whole weight is therefore taken on the sound leg. Therefore, when practising to stand up, the patient should be made to carry as much of his weight as possible on the affected leg. To this end his feet should be placed parallel or, better still, with the sound foot in front of the affected one before standing up. Even when this initial position of his feet is obtained before standing up, he may at the last moment pull the sound foot back automatically. This can be prevented by the therapist putting her foot lightly on the patient's foot. The patient is then encouraged to lean well forward at the hips, so that he starts putting weight on both his legs before he actually stands up. His arms should be stretched well forward and his hands clasped, and he should not look down. To begin with, the therapist can hold the patient's clasped hands to give some support and pull him forward and upward. She can also give some pressure on the patient's knee to reinforce his sensation of weightbearing and, at the same time, pull the knee a little forward to prevent sudden hyperextension and also the pushing backward of his hip with plantiflexion of the foot. In this way, he is made to take weight on the affected leg while it is still in some degree of flexion, and dorsiflexion of the ankle is maintained when he slowly extends knees and hips. Care should be taken to see that his trunk does not lean over towards the sound side. Sitting down is practised in the reverse way. It is useful if, as well as standing up and sitting down, he practises intermediate stages of the movement, i.e. standing up only a little way and going down again without actually sitting. When sitting down, it is the last stage which is most difficult for him to control as he tends to drop heavily on to his chair with his seat, but it is the most important. The height of the chair should be adjusted, starting with a fairly high one and progressing gradually to lower chairs or a low plinth. This is because standing up is more difficult from a low seat or chair and requires weightbearing on the flexed leg, which is a problem for all hemiplegic patients (Figs. 6.26a, b).

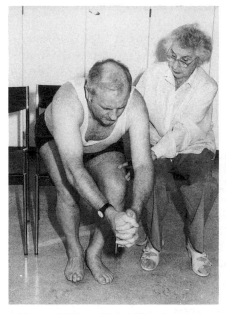

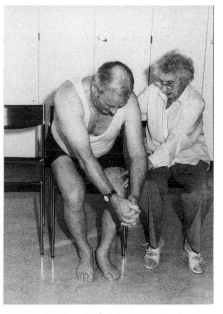

Fig. 6.26a Weightbearing on flexed legs.
Note: Affected foot is parallel with sound one.

Fig. 6.26b Starting to stand up. Weight on the affected leg.

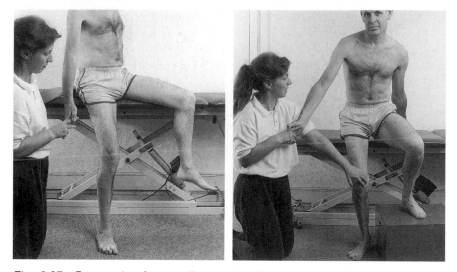

Fig. 6.27   Preparation for standing on the affected leg. (a) Getting down from plinth, taking weight on the affected leg. (b) Extension of hip and knee with foot firmly on the ground. The sound leg is flexed and not weightbearing.

Another way of helping the patient to stand up and take the full weight on the affected leg is to ask him to put his affected foot down to the ground from a high plinth while still sitting on the sound hip and supporting himself with the sound hand. His foot should touch the ground as near to the plinth as possible. This brings the whole of the affected side well forward, especially the pelvis and hip. In order to counteract extensor spasticity, the therapist keeps his foot in full dorsiflexion with one hand, while with her other she holds his hand supinated and keeps his elbow extended so that associated reactions, with increase of flexor spasticity, cannot occur. When the heel is well down on the ground, the patient is asked, and if necessary, helped, to extend his knee and keep it extended. In doing this, his hip also extends and, with encouragement, he may be able to lift his seat a fraction off the support. Hyperextension of the knees is prevented by the edge of the plinth, which keeps the pelvis well forward. In this way, he exercises the quadriceps and hip-extensors without extensor spasticity as his foot remains dorsiflexed. When he can keep his knee extended, he should practise small isolated movements of his knee, alternating flexion with extension. When he feels safe and has got the experience of weightbearing with controlled movements of his knee, he should lift the sound hand off the support to get more weight on the leg, and so become aware that it is strong enough for him to stand on it (Figs. 6.27a, b).

So far, he has been sitting, but now he is asked to put the sound leg down also and to place his foot parallel with the affected one. He is, at first, still allowed to lean against the plinth, but he should not hold on

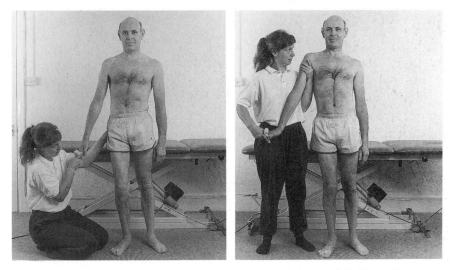

Fig. 6.28a Alternating flexion and extension of knee. (b) Therapist keeps shouldergirdle raised with arm and hand extended, and in external rotation inhibiting flexor spasticity.

to it. To begin with his weight should be equal on both legs. Weight transfer is then practised, with emphasis towards the affected side. Next the patient is asked to bend and extend both knees together followed by bending and extending first one and then the other. Usually, the patient finds the independent action of one leg from the other difficult, and he tends to bend both knees simultaneously. When he has mastered this difficulty, treatment is advanced towards reciprocal action, i.e. bending one knee while, at the same time, extending the other. This movement is essential for walking and is very important to obtain (Figs. 6.28a, b).

Up to now the patient has been allowed to lean against the plinth, which gave him security, as he did not need to balance. Now he is asked, and helped, to move his hips forward and away from the plinth. The therapist, having been in front of the patient before, now stands by his affected side. To begin with, she puts one arm across his lower back to help him to balance and to move his hips forward. He should keep his head up, because looking down makes extension of his hips difficult. When he feels safe standing away from the plinth and having his full weight on the affected leg, he is asked to lift the heel of the sound foot off the ground to start balancing on the affected leg. This is followed by making successive very small steps forward and backward with the sound foot. These steps should not only be short, but should also be done slowly, so that the patient maintains his full weight on the affected leg as long as possible. In this way, he also learns to transfer weight over the standing leg, bringing his pelvis forward with his hip extended. If this is not practised early on, he will

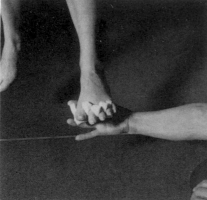

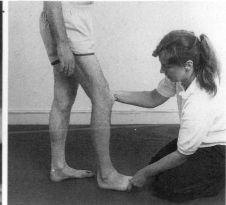

Fig. 6.29 Foam spreader for toes to inhibit plantar flexion and clawing of toes.

Fig. 6.30 Stepping foward with affected leg. Therapist controls pressure downwards of leg and foot. Note: In this way, control of extensor spasticity keeps knee mobile.

get used to making steps of unequal length, or he may make quick long steps with the sound leg and then drag the affected leg to the level of the sound foot. Some patients do the opposite. They make large steps with the affected leg, but then cannot transfer their weight far enough forward over the affected foot because of insufficient dorsiflexion. They then have to make a very quick short step with the sound foot to bring it to the level of the affected one.

Extensor spasticity interferes with dorsiflexion of the ankle and toes. In most patients we find excessive plantiflexion of the toes in standing and walking and, in some, the toes bend and curl right under the foot becoming painful. A 'toe-spreader' of foam rubber helps to separate the toes because their abduction counteracts plantiflexion and reduces extensor spasticity of the whole foot, and often of the entire leg (Fig. 6.29). If the therapist puts her hand under the ball of the patient's foot, she will find that there is strong pressure and that, in fact, the patient pushes against her hand. This pressure stiffens his knee and prevents dorsiflexion of ankle and toes. It is a great obstacle for the swing-phase of his leg in walking as he cannot release his knee and foot to make a step forward. It also interferes with weightbearing on the heel and with transfer of weight from heel to toes.

In treatment, therefore, the therapist places her hand under the ball of the patient's foot, lifts his toes and dorsiflexes his ankle while he stands on his heel. This is done until there is no pressure to be felt; then the front of his foot is gently lowered again to the ground and pressure downward prevented. Dorsiflexion then becomes possible at a greater range and the patient is asked to bring his weight well forward with his hip extended, as in transferring weight to make a step forward with his sound leg (Fig. 6.30). Hyperextension of the knee should be avoided.

Treatment for walking

Unfortunately, a short brace is prescribed for many patients who would not need one if dorsiflexion of the ankle and toes in standing, and weight transfer over the affected foot was practised early on in treatment, i.e. before the patient is made to walk. A brace may be necessary in patients who have much sensory loss and do not feel it when the ankle turns over. In some cases, there is no danger of the foot turning over and little spasticity of the leg, but active dorsiflexion of the ankle is impossible; the foot then drops rather than pushes down. In order to keep the ankle flexed, a back-splint, moulded to the calf of the leg, attached to a support in the shoe, is preferable to a short brace.

Though the patient may feel safer with a brace and may use one for a while for long stretches of walking out of doors, it has a number of disadvantages such as:

1. The patient who is more flaccid than spastic exhibits more flexor than extensor spasticity at hip and knees, although he cannot actively dorsiflex his ankle. The brace, keeping the foot in dorsiflexion, prevents sufficient extensor activity at knee and hip; the hip remains in some flexion and is unstable. To stabilize the knee, the patient locks it in hyperextension.
2. Balance at the ankle cannot develop, as activity and sensation of the ankle movement is limited, and muscle wasting is likely to occur.
3. Ankle clonus may be produced through stretch reflexes in patients whose spasticity is moderate or slight.

When walking with the patient, the therapist, nurse or relatives should never be on his sound side as the patient himself can balance and control his movements on that side. If balance and weight transfer have been practised in standing, and the patient is able to make short steps forward and backward with the sound leg, he should be able to manage with an ordinary walking stick and will not need a tripod or quadripod to lean on. (There are, however, a few exceptions to this, for example, very old patients and those with severe sensory loss on the affected side.) If the patient leans heavily on a tripod, his whole weight is on the sound arm and leg and his trunk leans over towards the tripod when making a step with the affected leg (Fig. 6.31). As he moves his leg forward with a stiff knee and circumduction of the hip, the affected side of his trunk shortens. The pull of the side-flexors of the trunk on the affected side when hitching the pelvis up reinforces the flexor spasticity of arm and hand. The therapist should not teach the patient to 'lock' his knee in the stance phase, as

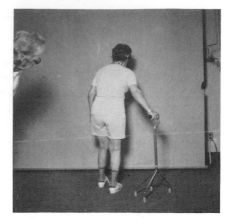

Fig. 6.31 Walking with tripod. Weight completely on sound side. Note: Shortening of involved side.

this will result in 'back-kneeing' and is difficult to correct later on. If he is made to extend his hip and bring it well forward, his knee also extends, but without hyperextension (Fig. 6.32). All the various phases of walking can be prepared for in standing. It should then be unnecessary to splint the knee, which prevents its flexion when making a step and thus makes circumduction a necessity. In a few cases, it may be preferable to teach the patient to walk with slightly flexed knees, but only as a temporary measure.

Gait training should be done from the beginning without letting the patient use a stick, so that he develops a symmetrical walking pattern with weightbearing on the affected leg. (However, the patient should be assisted by the therapist or nurse until he has sufficient balance and is in no danger of falling.) Many patients will then be able to walk without a stick, at least at home, although some may need one for safety when walking outdoors.

In order to prepare for a reasonably normal gait, balance, stance

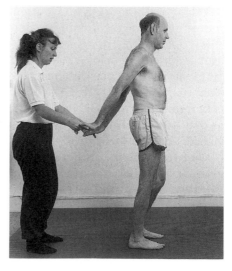

Fig. 6.32 Moving pelvis forward over affected right leg. This prevents hyperextension of knee. Note: Inhibition of flexor spasticity of arm. Patient moves trunk against limbs.

and weight transfer should be practised. For the swing phase, the patient needs release of spasticity at hip, knee and ankle to lift his leg and make a step. He also needs control of the extending leg when putting his foot down to the ground. If all this is first practised while in the standing position, he will develop a better walking pattern than if he is made to walk immediately without the necessary control of his leg. When analysing the patient's difficulties in walking, we find two main problems:

1. In the stance phase, we find excessive co-contraction of both extensor and flexor patterns inhibiting movement. This allows the patient to take weight on the affected leg momentarily, but makes the limb immobile and excludes all balance reactions. (Co-contraction of a moderate degree plays a normal role in our movements and is necessary for giving us stability to maintain posture against gravity, for giving fixation to moving parts, for weightbearing and, on the arm, for lifting and carrying weights.)
2. In the swing phase, moving the weightfree affected leg for making a step with a mobile knee so that he does not use circumduction at the hip with the pelvis pulled up on the affected side.

There are two types of patient

1. Those patients with both flexor and extensor spasticity, but predominant extensor hypertonus of the leg, i.e. excessive co-contraction. They can stand and take some weight for a moment when walking with a stiff leg. These patients have great problems with the swing-phase of walking.
2. By contrast, other patients with more moderate degrees of spasticity and little co-contraction can walk and move the weightfree leg, but only in a total pattern of flexion and extension. They may have a reasonably good swing phase, but cannot stand safely on the affected leg and, when weight-bearing, are unstable.

Both types of patient have balance problems, the first because of lack of mobility, and the other due to lack of stability. Therefore, if extensor spasticity is strong, the patient has more difficulty with the swing phase than with standing and weightbearing, though balance and weight-transfer are problems: his knee and foot are too stiff to make a step. Patients with only slight extensor spasticity, but with a tendency to flexion and abduction of the leg will find standing and weightbearing more problematical. These patients can easily lift the leg for a step, but tend to collapse on it when standing and lifting the sound leg for making a step. Both the stance and swing phases have to be well prepared before a good walking pattern can be obtained (Lane, 1978).

The stance phase

The patient tends to hold his leg stiffly extended and pushes with the ball of his foot and with his toes against the ground, which prevents dorsiflexion at the ankle to allow for weight transfer over the foot of the affected leg in walking. In order to keep his heel on the ground because of insufficient dorsiflexion, he hyperextends his knee and flexes his hip. His leg is stiff and, therefore, he cannot balance on it safely when he lifts the sound leg to step forward. Even when standing on both feet, he is afraid to transfer his weight from the sound leg to the affected one. He usually stands with his full weight on the sound leg, the affected one abducted and free of weight. Standing with his feet parallel and close together is difficult for him, but is his first means towards getting some weight on the affected leg.

In treatment, the patient is made to stand in front of the plinth, his feet close together. The therapist is by his affected side. With one hand she supports him under the axilla to keep his shouldergirdle raised, and with her other she supports his hand with wrist and elbow extended. The patient is then asked to move his hip towards her and helped to transfer his whole weight towards the affected side. When he feels safe, he is asked to make very small steps forward and backward with the sound leg. As he steps backward, his sound foot should move well behind the affected one. He should not bend his trunk forward and flex his hip, but keep it well extended, as this counteracts hyperextension of the knee. In this way, he learns to transfer weight over the standing leg and to control every phase of it.

When he is in step position, he is asked to maintain his full weight and to balance on the affected leg with the sound foot in front. He

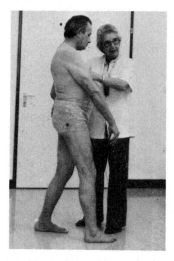

Fig. 6.33   Weightbearing and balancing of affected left leg with sound foot in front.

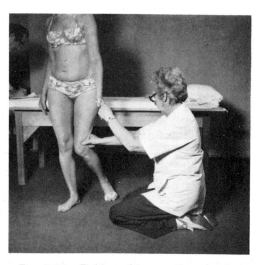

Fig. 6.34   Flexion of knee with extended hip without pulling pelvis upwards, prior to making a step forwards.

should then transfer his weight forward to the sound one, leaving the affected leg behind with the heel on the ground. His greatest balance problems occur when he has to have his full weight on the affected leg while the sound one remains in front: he tends to fall backwards if he flexes the hip of the weightbearing leg. Small isolated movements of the knee alternating flexion with extension should be practised to ensure mobility of the weightbearing leg (Fig. 6.33).

To obtain weightbearing with weight transfer and balance on the stance leg while walking, the patient steps forward and backwards, but only touches the ground lightly with his sound foot. The body weight remains on the affected leg while he transfers it forwards and backwards over the weightbearing leg. The same procedure can be used while the patient is walking by making him touch the ground lightly with the sound foot, once or twice, before he makes a step, and without putting any weight on that leg. In this way, firm weightbearing is maintained on the affected leg during weight transfer in walking.

The swing phase

When the patient's affected leg is stiff in extension and his foot pushes against the ground, it is difficult for him to bring it forward or backward to make a step without pulling up his pelvis and circumducting it. He should not be allowed to lift his leg high up as he can only do this by pulling up his pelvis. Instead, before making a step, he should be helped to release his knee and bend it slightly, with his pelvis lowered, and then to bring his flexed knee forward (Fig. 6.34). Selective movements of the knee have already been practised in standing on the affected leg, but bending his knee and keeping his hip extended when the affected leg is behind the sound one is more difficult for him. Hip extension with a flexed knee has been practised before in supine (Figs. 6.11a, b and Fig. 6.12b, pp. 95, 96), and should now be practised again with the leg lowered over the edge of the plinth, the hip fully extended and the knee made to bend. In the younger patient, where prone-lying is no problem, as it may be with the very old, it can also be done in prone. The therapist bends the patient's knee until there is no resistance to flexion. He is then asked to hold it flexed and to maintain it in various degrees of flexion when the leg is gradually extended by the therapist (placing) (Fig. 6.35).

The patient should now stand with his full weight on the sound leg, the affected one slightly behind it. He is asked to relax and bend his affected knee, adducting his thigh so that his knee comes near the sound one. His foot should remain on the ground in pronation. This gives him a pattern of adduction with the knee flexed and his pelvis lowered. The leg is now relaxed and in position to make a step forward (Fig. 6.36). When he starts to make a step, however, there may still be some pressure of the toes against the ground, which may

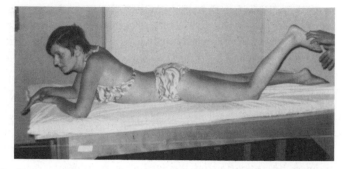

Fig. 6.35   Preparing flexion of knees with extended hip and dorsiflexion of ankle in preparation for walking without circumduction.

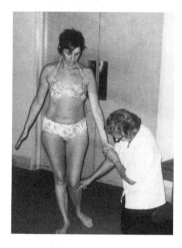

Fig. 6.36   Flexion of knee with hip extended and lowered to allow for step forward without circumduction. (Left leg affected)

produce supination of the ankle and stiffening of the knee. He then cannot release and bend the knee or dorsiflex the ankle and toes to make a normal step forward. He is forced to make a step with a stiff knee and plantiflexed foot. In order not to scrape the ground with his toes, he has to pull his pelvis upwards and circumduct his leg. The therapist, therefore, lifts his foot off the ground, just as much as the patient would have to do for making a step forward, and tests for resistance to this movement. She should then put his foot down again, asking him not to push it down. He is next asked to lift his foot without pulling his pelvis upwards, but as he does so, the therapist may have to control his foot and prevent supination.

The patient should also practise doing small alternating movements of flexion and extension of his knee, while keeping his toes on the ground (Figs. 6.37a, b). When he can do this without stiffening his knee, he should be asked to make a step forward. The therapist may guide his foot, controlling his dorsiflexed toes to prevent supination and pressure against the ground when he puts it down in front. As a progression, the same manouevre can be practised with the patient's

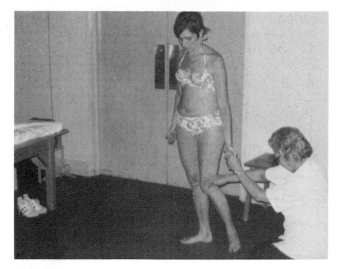

Fig. 6.37a   The patient performs small alternating movements of flexion and extension of the knee.

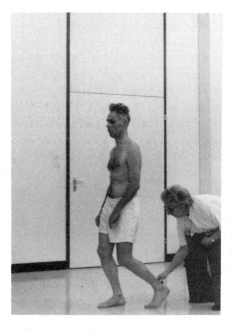

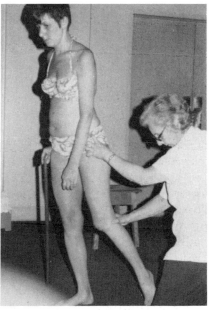

Fig. 6.37b   The control of dorsiflexion of the spastic left foot prior to making a step forward.

Fig. 6.37c   Flexion of knee of affected leg when it is further behind in preparation for making larger steps. Knee flexion of affected leg is more difficult because of increased hip extension with extensor spasticity. Pulling up of the pelvis is prevented by the therapist.

leg further behind the sound one, in the position he will need it for making a larger step. The release of extensor spasticity of the knee is then more difficult as the hip is fully extended and the toes are more likely to press against the ground (Fig. 6.37c).

When putting his foot down in front, the patient should learn to control the weight of his leg as he lowers it towards the ground. He should not drop his leg, but place his foot down gently. He must not stiffen his knee and foot when touching the ground, as this will produce plantiflexion and supination at the ankle and make heel-toe strike impossible. If his foot is stiff when touching the ground, full dorsiflexion for weight transfer over the now weightbearing leg will be impossible. Then, the tendo-achilles becomes tight and the patient hyperextends his knee. Some patients avoid the problem of putting the heel down by keeping the extended leg in external rotation and abduction at the hip. External rotation and abduction belong to the total flexor synergy and break up the total extensor synergy with adduction, and plantiflexion and supination of the foot. In this way, sufficient dorsiflexion with pronation of the foot becomes possible, so that the patient can put his heel down in spite of the knee remaining stiff in extension. However, circumduction and the pulling up of the pelvis will still be necessary in order to clear the ground, but it is undesirable as it tends to perpetuate the abnormal walking pattern.

Control of extensor spasticity of the leg has been practised before in supine and sitting, but now it is done in standing and walking. After the patient has moved his leg forward, leading with his knee and without lifting it any higher than would be done for a normal step, he should lower his foot down to the ground very slowly. It is useless to encourage the patient to lift his leg up high, for he would only use a total flexor pattern with great effort and his arm would flex and become more spastic. He would have to lower his leg by pushing his foot down in front, toes first, and would have difficulty in putting his heel down afterwards. In normal walking, we do not lift the leg up in front, but bring it forward, leading with a flexed knee and strong dorsiflexion of ankle and toes. The therapist, when asking the patient to make a step, controls the foot in dorsiflexion and checks whether there is any pressure of the foot against her hand (Fig. 6.38). When pressure is felt by the therapist, the patient is asked to lift the foot again for a moment before putting it down so that extensor spasticity can be inhibited. When the foot touches the ground without weight on it, he should perform isolated movements of his knee repeatedly to keep his leg mobile for making a step backwards, now leading with the heel. While his knee is mobile, he is asked to make very small steps forwards and backwards without taking weight on the leg and without pulling his hip up. If necessary, the therapist can hold his pelvis down on the affected side to facilitate independent movements of his knee. This procedure can be included into his walking pattern. The patient is then asked just to tip the ground lightly with the toes of the swing

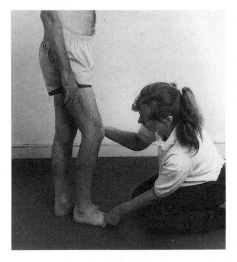

Fig. 6.38   Patient making step forward. Therapist controls and inhibits excessive spasticity with downward pressure of foot.

leg before he puts weight on it. In this way, he controls excessive extensor activity and keeps the leg free to move for the next step.

A good way of improving the patient's gait is to ask the patient to stand on a small base with his feet parallel, and rotate his pelvis, i.e. twist his trunk against his limbs, for a few seconds. This is followed by his making a few steps with improved coordination, after which the improved walking pattern will again deteriorate. He should then stand still again, and repeat the rotation of the pelvis before taking the next step. The affected side should come well forward during this rotation. Rotation inhibits the spastic pattern and gives the patient bilateral function instead of the asymmetrical pattern he has used previously. The two sides of his body then interact and do not act separately any longer.

It is usually easier for a patient to walk sideways on a line, if the therapist wants him to move his knee, than to walk forwards or backwards, especially if he walks sideways towards the sound side. The advantage when walking sideways towards the affected side is that he has to take full weight on to that leg. However, she should make sure that the patient does not place the affected foot in front of the line.

Treatment in prone-lying and kneeling

Since writing the second edition of this book, I have found that treatment in prone and kneeling is of limited value in the older patients with hemiplegia, many of whom have circulatory problems and cannot tolerate prone-lying. Kneeling is often uncomfortable or painful for those who have arthritis and stiff joints, or for those who are very heavy and would probably have difficulty in getting down on the floor and up again even without hemiplegia. Much of the benefit which can be obtained in prone and kneeling can also be obtained in the more functional activities of daily life, for instance, forearm support and movements of the elbow and hand can be practised while sitting at a table, and extended arm support while standing in front of a wall or table.

It is important, however, that, if possible, all patients be taught how to get up from the floor in case they should fall at any time. They should learn to sit up towards the unaffected side, to get up to half-kneeling with the sound foot forward, and to reach for a support with the sound hand, and so to stand up. Treatment in four-foot kneeling, kneel-standing and half-kneeling will help in practising to stand up from the floor and will make the patient less afraid of falling. Treatment in kneeling is also important for weightbearing on the affected leg without the use of the total extensor synergy; it helps towards the use of the arm and hand in extension for support and balance. However, in kneeling the treatment is useful only for younger and more mobile patients. The patient is taught to get down on to his hands and knees by first bending the affected leg and immediately putting weight on it. The affected arm should, if necessary, be supported, the elbow held in extension and the hand placed flat on the ground with the fingers extended and the thumb abducted. The weight of the body should be well over the affected arm and leg. He is then made to rock forward and backward and from side to side, in order to obtain mobility and balance reactions. Later on, the sound leg or arm is lifted and the patient has to support his weight mainly on the affected side (Figs. 6.39a, b).

From four-foot kneeling, the patient is encouraged to raise his head and trunk so that he stands on his knees only. However, it is often

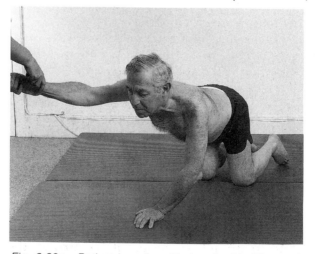

Fig. 6.39a   *Patient kneeling. He is asked to lift sound arm.*
Note: *Poor balance and arm support on left affected side.*

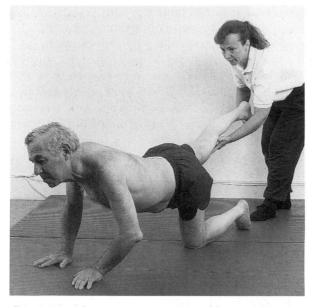

Fig. 6.39b   Rocking backwards and forward, balancing on affected knee.

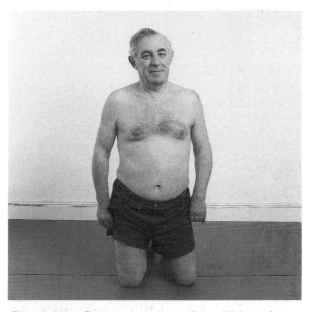

Fig. 6.39c   Patient kneel-standing. Weight is on affected side, but note slight retraction of affected side.

difficult for him to get full extension of his hips in this position, especially of the affected hip, and there is also a tendency for him to put less weight on the affected leg than on the sound one (Fig. 6.39c). In order to help him to get full extension, the patient's arms are first elevated in external rotation, and then his hands are placed on the therapist's shoulders as she stands in front of him. She then stands by his affected side and moves the affected arm down to his side, held in extension at the elbow, his hand being supported and his wrist fully extended. Weight transfer is then practised from side to side, the therapist moving the patient's body as far as possible towards the affected side in order to encourage balance reactions of the affected leg. This procedure can also be practised with the patient as he stands

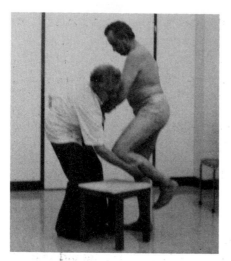

Fig. 6.40a   Therapist helps to place patient's knee on stool. (Left side affected)

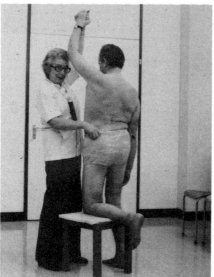

Fig. 6.40b   Extension of hip with flexed knee on stool.

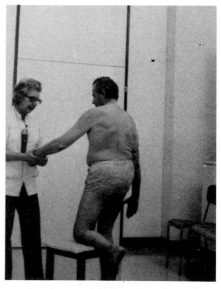

Fig. 6.40c   Making small steps forward and backwards with sound leg, while affected leg remains on stool. Note: *This movement practises weightbearing on affected hip.*

by the side of a chair or stool with his affected knee resting on the seat. This makes extension of the hip, and also weightbearing on the affected hip, easier than in kneel-standing on the floor. To obtain full weightbearing and balance, the patient is asked to make small steps forward and backward with the sound leg. Increase of flexor-spasticity of the arm should be prevented by controlling his elbow and wrist in extension either at his side or above his head (Figs. 6.40a, b, c).

Treatment in the second stage for control of movements of the arm

At this stage, the patient still has great difficulty in lifting and holding his arm up against gravity, because flexor spasticity of the trunk and shouldergirdle with pressure downwards prevents the action of the extensors, i.e. serratus anterior, deltoid and supraspinatus. Inhibition of spasticity can be achieved more easily in supine, as already described in the first stage of treatment (p. 103) and this has to be continued in preparation for working in the upright posture. It is easily obtained in standing, rather than in sitting, because in standing extension of the hips facilitates lifting of the arm whereas, in sitting, flexion of the hips and trunk make inhibition of flexor spasticity more difficult.

In order to make lifting of the arm possible, the patient must first be able to hold it at various stages when lowering it. He should extend his elbow and keep it extended all the way down. But extension alone is not sufficient. The arm should be in external rotation and supination, as internal rotation and pronation are part of the flexor pattern which counteracts lifting and holding the arm up. Control for holding the arm up at the shoulder is easier when it is held sideways rather than forward and down. This is because extension with external rotation and supination can be maintained more easily sideways than forward.

In supine, standing and sitting, it is easier for the patient to hold his arm against gravity than to lift it up. If he can control the weight of his arm all the way downward, he can also learn to lift it up from any downward point at which he is able to hold it. If the arm pulls down at any stage of the downward movement, the therapist will feel downward pressure against her support (which should be very light) and the movement should then immediately be reversed upward, either by the therapist or, better if possible, by the patient. He soon learns to recognize the moment when flexor spasticity occurs and his elbow tends to bend. To begin with, the therapist holds the patient's hand with wrist and fingers extended, the thumb abducted. The patient extends his elbow, pushing against the therapist's hand. She should be able to use some intermittent pressure to stimulate active extension. When he can hold his elbow in full extension, she moves his hand slowly sideways and down, but only as long as he is able to keep his elbow extended. He is then asked to move his arm up again. Gradually, the whole range of movement sideways for full horizontal abduction is performed. The movement is then done diagonally forward, as long as external rotation can be maintained. As a progression, the therapist holds the patient's fingers, but only lightly, to prevent the occurrence of flexion until, eventually, she is able to take her hand away at various points of the downward movement, and the patient is able to control his arm at each stage. This is called 'placing'. At which ever point the patient can arrest the downward movement, he should be able to lift his arm up from that point. Movement straight forward and down while holding and controlling the arm is more difficult and should be done with the patient's shoulder kept well forward, avoiding internal rotation. Full external rotation and supination, however, will be impossible for a long time, although it should be the ultimate aim (Figs. 6.41a, b, c, d).

If the patient's arm is more flaccid than spastic, contraction of the deltoid, for holding the arm up in horizontal abduction, can be facilitated by suddenly and without warning dropping the arm, but letting it fall only a little way down, and then moving it up again. Letting it fall may produce a protective holding reaction through sudden stretch in the inner range of the deltoid and supraspinatus. The patient can then use this contraction immediately, i.e. before its effect has subsided, for lifting his arm up again. This manoeuvre will not work, however, if there is any flexor spasticity.

Another way of stimulating active extension of the flaccid arm is a technique which we call 'pull-push'. With the patient's hand held with wrist and fingers extended, his arm is raised sideways to the horizontal, or above, and a quick pull, followed by a push against his extended arm, is given through his hand. This stimulates mobile extension of the elbow and a holding action at the shoulder. The patient now feels that he can extend his arm without it stiffening, and

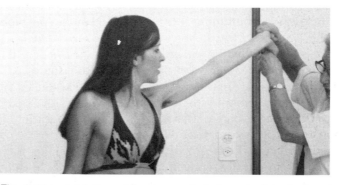

Fig. 6.41a *Inhibition of flexor spasticity to make 'placing' and holding of arm possible. Patient moves trunk backwards, forwards and sideways.*

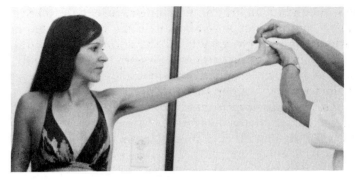

Fig. 6.41b   *When resistance of wrist flexors has been reduced, abduction of thumb with extension of fingers only is needed.*

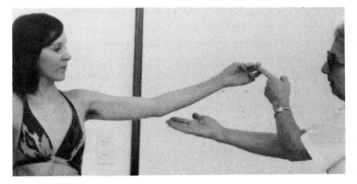

Fig. 6.41c   *After successful inhibition of flexor spasticity, the position of the arm can be actively maintained with little support by the therapist. 'Placing' is now possible.*

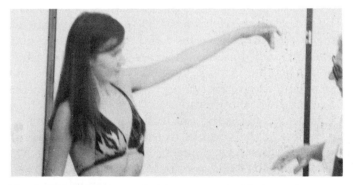

Fig. 6.41d   *Patient now holds up arm unaided.*
Note: *However, she is not yet able to maintain the arm in external rotation.*

through the pull, followed quickly by pushing against the extended arm, the therapist inhibits flexor spasticity. This combination of inhibition and stimulation is very useful and should be done with the patient's arms in any direction, sideways, forward and diagonally, and also gradually downwards. When sufficient activation has been obtained at shoulder and elbow, the therapist lets go of the patient's hand and he should hold his arm up unaided.

Inhibition of flexor spasticity has to be done during and, if necessary, in between all the 'placing' manoeuvres described above, i.e. when the patient's arm becomes heavy and uncontrolled, or when a pull downwards is noticed by the therapist.

The patient may now be able to lift and hold his arm at the shoulder, provided he keeps his elbow extended. The moment he is asked to bend his elbow so that he can bring his hand to his body or face, the whole pattern of flexion, pronation and downward pressure of the side-flexors of his trunk and retraction of his shouldergirdle may come into play, and he can no longer hold his arm up. For functional use, i.e. for feeding, dressing and other activities, it is essential that he should be enabled to bend and supinate his elbow and open his hand to grasp, while holding and stabilizing his raised arm at the shoulder. Treatment, therefore, should be advanced towards obtaining independent movements of the elbow without letting the arm fall.

Working for independent and controlled movements of the elbow

Controlled movements of the elbow are practised at first with the upper arm still supported. Flexion of the elbow, even with supination, does not usually present a problem for the patient as it is done with flexor spasticity, but the return to extension is difficult or impossible. In supine, or sitting, the patient is now able to hold his arm up extended above his head. He is asked to bend his elbow to touch the top of his head with his palm without dropping his arm at the shoulder, followed by moving his hand to the opposite shoulder, then back again to his head and up above his head. He can also be made to touch the opposite ear and then move his hand to the shoulder and down the arm, as if washing himself. Whenever he moves his hand downwards, he should be able to raise it again. He should keep his shoulder well forward and any retraction of the shouldergirdle must be prevented, if necessary by the therapist supporting his shoulder from behind and holding it forward. She can also put her fingers against the medial aspect of the scapula and mobilize it in a lateral direction to counteract the patient's tendency to fix it medially.

Independent movements of the elbow can also be practised with the patient lying on his affected side, his arm extended and in full external rotation. Again, his shoulder should be placed well forward. He is then asked to bend his elbow to bring his hand to his mouth, and then back to extend it again. This movement of the elbow should be slow and controlled at every stage, as the forearm tends to pronate and fall when about 90° of flexion has been reached. If it does, he may not be able to extend the elbow again. The same movements can be practised in supine with the patient's arm lying in horizontal abduction, or lower down by his side. He should then touch his shoulder with his supinated hand (*see* Figs, 6.8a, b, p. 91). In sitting, it is best practised with the forearm resting on a table, the shoulder held well forward to avoid the usual pattern of elbow flexion with retraction at the shoulder. Flexion of the elbow with supination brings his hand to his mouth and to the opposite shoulder or ear. In fact, he learns to control movements which he needs for the functional use of his hand later on. His hand should remain open and internal rotation with pronation, which tends to occur when the elbow is fully flexed, should be avoided.

So far the patient's upper arm has been supported and stabilized by the table, but he should gradually practise the above-described selective movements of the elbow while he holds and controls the arm at the shoulder (Figs. 6.42a, b).

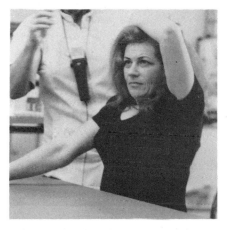

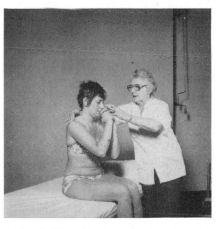

Fig. 6.42a Independent movements of elbow while holding arm up
at shoulder.

Fig. 6.42b Moving clasped hands
to face.
Note: Therapists's right hand prevents retraction of shoulder.

Exercises the patient should do at home

Before the patient leaves hospital, a relative should be well instructed and trained with regard to his general management as well as being able to help him with his exercises.

The following exercises can eventually be done by the patient without the help of the therapist, and should be done at home as often as possible during the day to supplement treatment. They have to be part of treatment and only those which the patient can do well by himself should be done at home.

The patient clasps his hands and interlocks his fingers, with the thumb of the affected hand over that of the sound one, to ensure as much abduction of the thumb as possible. His wrist should be in semisupination and extended. Pronation of the affected forearm must be avoided. In sitting, or standing, he moves his hands above his head (Fig. 6.43). The elbows must be at the same level and the affected arm should not pull forward at the shoulder. This is followed by putting his clasped hands behind his head and then raising them again. Next, he puts his clasped hands on his chest, making sure that the affected arm does not pull backwards or drop down. From having his hands on his chest, he extends his arms forward so that his hands touch a wall or, if possible, a mirror on the wall. The affected arm tends always to be lower than the sound one because of depression of the shoulder, and this should be counteracted. If he finds this difficult, he should lift his arms up again above his head and bend his trunk sideways towards the sound side in order to release the downward pull of the side flexors of the affected side of his trunk and shouldergirdle. Then, he should again move his extended arms forward against a wall, and he will now find that it is easier to hold the affected arm up at the same level as the sound one.

Exercises with clasped hands to improve extension of wrist and fingers can be done by the patient turning his clasped hands so that the palms face forward, the back of his hands against his chest. He then extends his arms above his head, back to his chest, and forward against a mirror or wall (Figs. 6.44a, b). Shoulders and elbows should be level. With his hands now flat against the wall, he slides them up and down and sideways towards the sound side, the latter to help the forward movement of his affected shoulder. While standing, he can also place his hands down on a table and support himself on them.

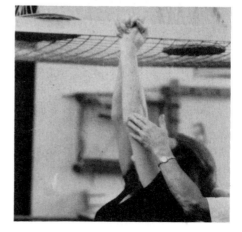

Fig. 6.43 Elevation of arms with clasped hands prior to placing hands on head.
Note: *Therapist holds up the upper arms while patient bends elbow.*

Keeping his hands on the table, he walks backwards to obtain a good stretch of his trunk with his shoulders forward, and he then walks forward again, still supported on his hands (Fig. 6.44c). When he can do this with his hands clasped, he can practise standing in front of a wall with his open hands placed flat against it. When doing this in treatment, the therapist should help him to abduct his thumb and spread his extended fingers (at home, to begin with, he can do this with the sound hand). Then he bends and extends his elbows, his hands remaining extended against the wall (Fig. 6.45). When he is

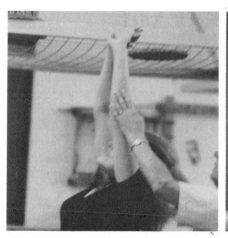

Fig. 6.44a With raised arms, patient turns clasped hands so that the palms face upwards and forward.

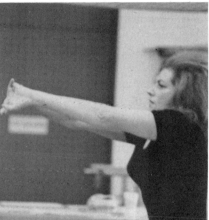

Fig. 644b The same movement with arms forward.

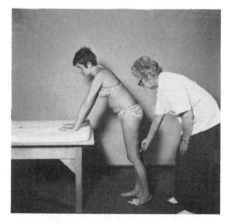

Fig. 6.44c Walking backwards while keeping palms on table, either with hands clasped or palms down.

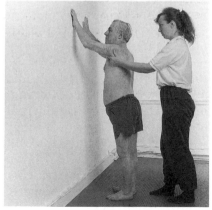

Fig. 6.45 Standing with arms raised and hands against the wall with palms flat.
Note: Therapist supports arm at shoulder, preventing pressure downwards.

able to keep his affected hand against the wall, he can turn his sound side away from it, the affected hand remaining on the wall, the elbow extended and the arm in horizontal abduction, in this way actively inhibiting flexor spasticity.

There are infinite variations of the above techniques which the therapist can invent and which will make treatment for the patient more interesting.

STAGE OF RELATIVE RECOVERY

The patients who reach the third stage of relative recovery will be those who were not severely affected at the beginning and who have made a good spontaneous recovery, or who have done well in treatment. These patients will now be able to walk unaided, i.e. without using a stick, to use the affected arm for support and to hold an object in the hand if it is placed into it. They may, however, be unable to use the hand for manipulation or have difficulty in doing so. It is desirable that these patients, who are able to work and to lead an independent life in the community, should be further helped by improving the quality of their gait and by obtaining better use of the affected hand.

It may be fairly easy to obtain improvement in walking and balance, and also in the use of the hand for simple grasp and release and as a 'support' for the sound hand. However, in many patients isolated use of the fingers, and especially of the thumb and index finger, may be unobtainable. Even if there should be a recovery of independent finger movements, sensory deficit may make the patient 'forget' his hand, so that he uses it only when he thinks about it and not automatically, as is normal.

Spasticity is slight at this stage and does not, therefore, prevent movement. Transient increase of spasticity, however, still occurs when the patient uses effort, walks fast, or gets excited; coordination then deteriorates. His knee and foot become stiff and flexion of his arm and hand increases and makes the use of the fingers for manipulation difficult, clumsy and slow. For instance, he may be able to move individual fingers and even oppose thumb to index finger without holding or manipulating an object and without holding his arm up against gravity. However, when trying to use the same movements with voluntary effort for a skill, his fingers will flex and become stiff. In most patients, small localized movements of the elbow, wrist and fingers, and of the knee, ankle and toes are impossible. Although the patient can bend and extend his leg, he bends it with a total pattern of flexion and abduction, and he extends it with adduction and internal rotation and plantiflexion of ankle and toes. He may be able to dorsiflex his ankle and toes when he bends his leg, but not when the leg is extended. His limbs will function too much in total patterns. There is a lack of selective movement and of the necessary variety and different combinations of movement of parts of the original, abnormal total pattern. The dissociation, i.e. the breaking up of total synergies not only makes selective movements possible, but also the resynthesis of such movements into new and different functional patterns. In a lecture on spasticity the Neurologist, Dr Denis Williams, explained the role of inhibition in producing an isolated movement. He said:

> 'In order to beckon someone to you with your index finger, do not think that you just contract your flexor indicis proprius—you inhibit the flexion of your whole arm.'

In treatment, the practice of inhibition for the performance of selective movements is done by preventing movements at other joints if and when the patient moves his elbow, his wrist or fingers, or his ankle and toes.

Treatment to improve the patient's gait

If further improvement in the patient's gait is to be achieved, it is necessary to obtain still more selective movements of his knee, and of dorsiflexion and plantiflexion of ankle and toes, independent of the position and movement of his hip. Full dorsiflexion of ankle and toes is essential for normal walking and for heel-toe strike. It is also necessary for balance in standing on the affected leg as a protective

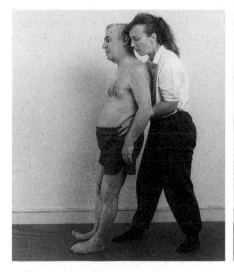

Fig. 6.46a Moving patient backwards.
Note: *Normal dorsiflexion of sound right foot (normal balance reaction, and its absence in affected foot).*

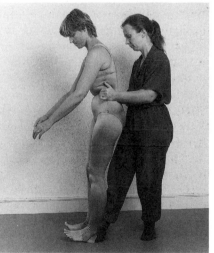

Fig. 6.46b Normal person moved backwards.
Note: *Dorsiflexion of ankles and toes; arms move forward as well as head.* See: *Equilibrium reactions, p. 43.*

postural reaction against falling backwards (Figs. 6.46a, b). Until this reaction has been obtained in treatment, we cannot expect or aim for heel-toe strike and the therapist should be satisfied when the patient can put his whole foot safely down to the ground—just as children do before they know how to put their heel down first.

In walking, more than 90° of dorsiflexion of the ankle is needed for sufficient weight transfer forward over the standing leg. This is practised in step-position with the sound foot well forward and the patient moving his hip as far as possible forward over the foot of the sound leg. He should keep the heel of the affected leg down on the floor (Fig. 6.47). The patient should then release his knee, bending it and moving it forward; as his heel leaves the ground, his toes should remain and become fully dorsiflexed. Here, the therapist may have to help in order to avoid supination of the foot, which happens if the patient pushes against the ground. This movement is then reversed, the patient putting his heel back again on to the ground; he should not push it down, but gently release his calf muscles and hip flexors so that his hip remains forward and extended. These alternate movements should be done a few times and then, when there is no extensor spasticity and no pressure of the toes against the ground, he should make a step forward. The therapist may still have to control the foot in dorsiflexion and pronation. He should lead with his knee and keep his hip lowered, and he should make small steps forward and backward. Stepping backward is done with his heel leading and no pressure should be felt by the therapist who controls the dorsiflexed foot.

The leg can also be kept mobile for the swing phase by letting the patient put his affected foot on a small trolley fitted with castors, and practising rolling it with movements of his hip and knee forward, sideways and backwards. The whole foot should remain on the trolley. This gives the patient a feeling of how to move his leg when making steps and prevents undesirable pressure downwards (Figs. 6.48a, b). The trolley can also be moved with the sound foot in order to improve balance reactions on the affected leg when standing. In addition, the trolley can be used to obtain independent movements of the patient's knee in sitting, especially by moving the trolley backwards towards the chair.

The patient himself can learn to check up and control any pressure he exerts with the affected leg by putting his affected foot on a pair of flat scales placed in front of him. He should watch and see that there is little or no weight shown on the scales. The scales are then placed diagonally forward and sideways so that he learns to make controlled steps in different directions. He should put his foot on and off the scales very slowly. The same manoeuvre can be practised standing on the affected leg and putting the sound foot on the scales slowly and lightly, so that the patient has to balance on the affected leg. Two flat scales can also be used, one for each foot, so that the patient can see

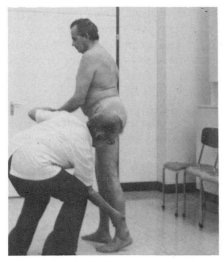

Fig. 6.47 Working for dorsiflexion of the affected foot while patient steps forward with sound leg.

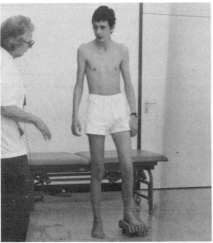

Fig. 6.48a Moving a small trolley backward with affected leg.

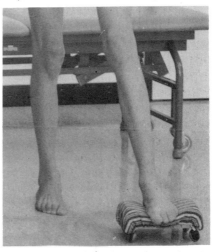

Fig. 6.48b Moving trolley forward.

and control how much weight he puts on each leg. When control of the swing phase has improved, the patient is asked to walk, but instead of immediately taking weight on the affected leg, he is asked to tip the ground lightly and quickly with his toes. He then immediately lifts his foot again to make a proper step and to put weight on the leg. This 'tipping' prevents undue pressure of the foot against the ground and, with it, stiffening of the knee. It is even better to let the patient do this tipping not only once between steps, but repeatedly. It can also be practised with the sound foot. It makes the patient stand and balance for longer periods on the affected leg than he would do otherwise (Fig. 6.49a). The movement should be confined to his hip and knee, and his pelvis should not pull upwards. When he can move his knee freely, he should bring the foot gradually backwards behind the sound one as in stepping backwards. Tipping the ground with the sound foot stops the patient from making quick steps with the sound leg in order to avoid weightbearing and weight transfer on the affected one and, instead, makes him take weight and balance on the affected leg.

To improve balance reactions on the affected leg, the therapist transfers the patient's weight well over to that leg. She stands by this side and holds his hand with his arm abducted and extended. His shouldergirdle should be prevented from pulling downward (Figs. 6.49a, b). He should be encouraged to flex his head laterally towards the sound side and his arm and leg on that side should lift and abduct. When he can do this well, he should be asked to perform small alternate movements of flexion and extension of the knee of the affected leg.

'Crossed' standing and walking is another way of improving his balance and the control of his hips, and is a preparation for rotation of the pelvis in walking. It also helps turning round towards the sound side, which the patient finds difficult, as he cannot bring the affected side sufficiently well forward (Figs. 6.50a, b).

When standing with his legs crossed, they should be externally rotated so that the toes of his feet point towards each other. When the affected leg is in front, his hip is extended and brought well forward. Small movements of his hips from side to side, or with rotation, can be done when he is safe enough to stand still and balance. He is then asked to bring the sound foot forward and across the affected one. He should do this slowly so that he carries his full weight for as long as possible on the affected leg. The therapist must guard against hyperextension of the knee at the back, which can be done by bending it a little to touch the back of the sound knee. The patient should then bring the affected leg forward again and across the sound one, but he should not abduct it more than absolutely necessary. This movement is very useful, as he has to bend his knee to get the affected leg in front of the sound one without circumducting the hip.

Walking backwards and forwards should be practised alternately by making, for instance, a few steps backwards and then one or two steps forward. When making a step backwards, the patient has to bend his knee and then he need not pull his pelvis upward. Walking backwards, therefore, improves walking forwards. As soon as the toes touch the ground at the back, he should gradually put his heel down before he puts weight on the leg. He should keep his hip well forward in extension; this prevents hyperextension of the knee and gives full dorsiflexion of the ankle (Fig. 6.51). Weight transfer forward and backward is practised in between making steps.

When walking, the therapist is at the patient's affected side. His arm is held in external rotation and extended by his side, slightly diagonally backwards. His wrist and fingers should be extended and

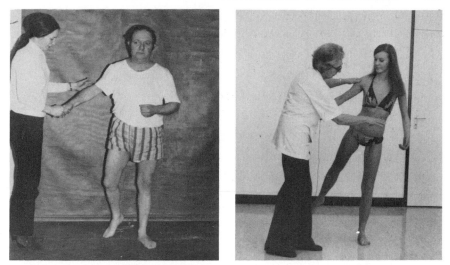

Figs. 6.49a, b   *Weightbearing and balance reactions facilitated on affected side.*

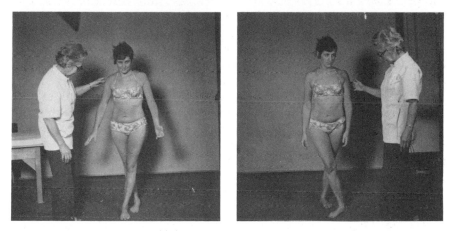

Figs. 6.50a, b   *Standing with legs crossed for weightbearing of affected leg and balance reactions.*
Note: *Rotation of pelvis practised.*

his thumb abducted. Walking can also be practised with the therapist behind the patient, holding both arms backward as described when sitting on a stool (p. 101, Figs. 6.16a, b). The patient then walks and moves his hip well forward over his foot before he makes a step with the sound leg (Fig. 6.52). When his weight is on the sound leg, he should stop for a moment before making a step with the affected one, so that he has time to release his knee, drop his pelvis on the affected side, and stop himself from pushing his foot down to the ground. He can then take a step forward.

Rotation of the pelvis and shouldergirdle is necessary practice to improve coordination in walking. Rotation of the shouldergirdle

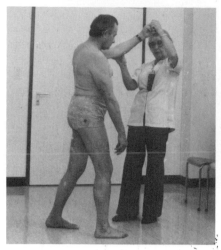 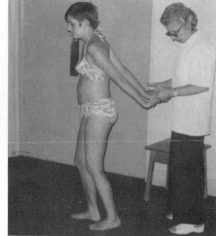

Fig. 6.51   Stepping backwards with affected left leg; getting heel to ground; balancing and weight transfer to affected leg.

Fig. 6.52   Walking with arms held backwards in extension. This helps towards extension of hip before making a step with sound leg.

makes arm swinging possible. Rotation of the pelvis inhibits spasticity of the leg by counteracting both total flexor and extensor patterns. It produces a normal interplay between the two sides of the body. Without rotation the patient moves the whole of the sound side forward and then drags the affected one to follow, i.e. he moves first with one side and then, to a lesser degree, with the other. This separation of the two sides is avoided by rotation as the two sides interact and alternate. With rotation, the 'dipping down' of the shouldergirdle and the pulling up of the pelvis is lessened and often disappears. Also, when the patient's shoulder is rotated backwards just before he puts his foot down to make a step, supination of the foot can be prevented (Fig. 6.53a).

Rotation of the shouldergirdle can first be practised by the patient in standing. He swings his arms from side to side rotating his trunk and touching the opposite thigh with one hand. To practise the same movement when walking, the therapist stands in front of the patient and holds him by both hands while she walks backwards. As the patient steps forward with, say, the right leg, she swings both his arms diagonally towards the right, the left arm well forward and across his body so that he touches his right thigh. As the patient transfers his weight over the right leg and makes a step with the left foot, the therapist reverses the movement of his arms. The rhythmical swinging of the arms and the rotation of his trunk helps to develop a more normal walking pattern. The movement of his arms have to be well timed to coincide with the patient's steps. The patient then continues this procedure unaided.

Another, and even better, way of introducing rotation into the patient's walking pattern can be done by the therapist standing behind him and rotating his hips or shouldergirdle. If she wants to influence the movement of his legs, it is better to rotate his pelvis; if she wants to work for more arm swinging, she rotates the shouldergirdle. The therapist should avoid bringing one side forward as a whole against the other (Figs. 53a, b, c). The patient should then perform rotation of the pelvis when standing without the help of the therapist and continue the movement when walking. However, if he

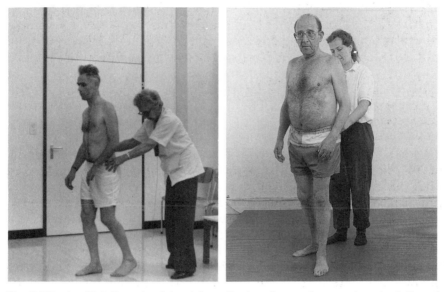

Fig. 6.53a, b   *Rotation of pelvis while patient walks produces external rotation of both legs and improves balance and walking patterns.*

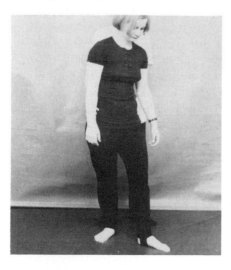

Fig. 6.53c   *Rotation of pelvis back-ward on left side facilitates external rotation of leg with everted foot.*

reverts to his former pattern of walking, i.e. moving one whole side against the other, he should stand still again, twisting his pelvis a few times before walking again.

The Integration of Physiotherapy and Occupational Therapy During the Third Stage

Treatment of the arm and hand

The treatment for the second (spasticity) and third (relative recovery) stages overlap and much of what has been done before should be continued, together with the practice of other activities which may now become possible. In these stages, close cooperation between the physiotherapist and the occupational therapist is of vital importance in order to ensure that there is carry-over of what the patient learns in physiotherapy into what is practised in occupational therapy, and from there into daily life. This is especially so with regard to the bilateral use of the arms and hands and, in some cases, with the use of the affected hand for independent grasp and release, regardless of the position or movement of the arm at the shouldergirdle and at the elbow. The patient's problems must be evaluated in the same way by the physiotherapist and the occupational therapist. The occupational therapist should understand the principles and ways of treatment used by the physiotherapist and vice versa. If the two disciplines work separately with different aims and in different ways, there is a great danger that they will work at cross purposes. The occupational therapist may then reinforce abnormal movement patterns and increase spasticity which the physiotherapist is trying to prevent. On the other hand, the physiotherapist may not know what the patient is expected to learn to do in occupational therapy and cannot, therefore, prepare for and include these activities in her treatment. The patient has to learn to move in different and more normal ways by the repetition of the same, or at least similar, activities.

As a first step toward good cooperation, they should make the first assessment of a patient together. Later, from time to time, reassessments will be found to be necessary. They should exchange ideas about treatment and find out, for example, what he might be able to do next in occupational therapy after having been prepared for it in physiotherapy. Specific problems should be discussed and ways of overcoming them tried out together.

In treatment, the occupational therapist should avoid causing effort and stress. It has been mentioned repeatedly that any effort, especially voluntary effort, increases spasticity. This then shows itself in stereotyped abnormal patterns which are useless for funtional skills. Even if the arm and hand are mobile at rest, they become stiff when the patient makes an effort to use them. Spasticity of the affected arm increases not only through effort in using the affected hand, but also through effort when using the sound one, and associated reactions and their abnormal patterns are then produced.

In those cases where the patient is unable to use his arm or hand, the occupational therapist should, to begin with, help him to become as independent as possible by teaching him self-help by the use of his sound hand alone. (In some cases, regrettably, a patient may have to rely on his sound hand indefinitely.) This is unfortunate as it produces and increases spasticity throughout the whole of the affected side. After a time, this could lead to a complete negation of the affected arm and hand by the patient. He will then never look at his arm and hand and ignore them. His arm will simply hang by his side, or he will tuck his hand under the table where he cannot see it. However, even if the patient's hand has no potential functional use, his trunk and arm must be trained for bilateral activity. This is why it is so important in the early stages for the patient to be made aware of his arm and hand and learn to feel and recognize them as part of himself. It will be impossible for him to achieve this later on if the sound arm and hand have been allowed to be used exclusively. At all times, therefore, his affected arm and hand should be in front of his body where he can see them and not hang helplessly by his side. In sitting, his weight should be well on the affected hip and in standing, for instance, at the work bench or blackboard, sink or washbasin, his weight should be on the affected leg. If complete orientation towards the sound side as a whole is encouraged at the beginning and for any length of time afterwards, the affected limbs will lose both sensory and motor potential. If a patient is able to grasp an object, he will do so by using flexor spasticity and then have great difficulty releasing it. This makes even the simplest function impossible. Again, if a patient is able to use his affected hand and is asked to do so for a task, he immediately becomes stressed and gets excited. He doubts whether he can do the required movement, he tries and may not succeed, or he may perform small clumsy movements with great effort. Stress and excitation in their turn increase spasticity and make the movement more difficult or impossible, thus producing a vicious circle. The occupational therapist, therefore, instead of asking for a 'voluntary' movement, should first work for a more 'automatic' movement of the same or similar pattern, i.e. for a movement which occurs without the patient having to 'think' about it. This can best be done in play, as a gesture when he speaks, with music or rhythm, or when asking him to count. Sometimes the automatic movement may be elicited by the therapist holding the patient's sound hand for a moment to prevent him from initiating the movement so that the patient uses the affected one first, and more automatically.

The manipulation of any object needs a great variety and many different combinations of selective movements. Movements of the hand should become independent of the position of the arm at the shoulder and elbow. The patient should learn to open and close his fingers and to oppose his thumb and fingers regardless as to whether the arm is elevated, abducted, flexed forward or hanging down by his side. He should be taught how to do this with the elbow extended or flexed, in supination and pronation. The movement patterns of arm and hand may still show a predominance of flexion with pronation of the forearm. All movements requiring flexion of the arm and hand in pronation are, therefore, fairly easy for the patient, while movements requiring supination, extension and abduction of thumb and fingers are more difficult. He can usually extend and move the outer three fingers, but the thumb and index finger remain stiff in flexion and he cannot use them. A patient may well be able to reach out and grasp a spoon, but have difficulty in bringing it to his mouth in supination. If he tries to do this, his fingers may open and he will lose his grasp. Grasp is often possible with a flexed elbow in pronation, and release only with supination and extension of the elbow. It is relatively easy to make a patient carry and hold an object with his elbow flexed and pronated, but when his arm is extended above his head, his hand will open and he can no longer hold the object. It is not only the position of the arm at the elbow and shoulder that determines and limits the use of his hand for holding and releasing an object: a patient, for instance, may well be able to lift his extended arm above his head and hold a brush, but when he bends his elbow to use it, he either cannot move his arm to brush his hair or, when he tries to move, he loses his grip of the brush. These difficulties are due to his inability to 'dissociate' the total patterns of flexion or extension and to combine various fragments of both patterns by inhibiting movements which do not belong to the intended activity.

Fog and Fog (1963) say:

> 'Cerebral inhibition serves the economy of cerebrospinal functional display. Through special inhibitory actions, primitive reflexes are suppressed or subordinated to higher level reflexes and reactions. So progressive cerebral inhibition promotes the coordinated adjustment of the body to internal and external stimuli. It is essential for the development of detailed, discriminate activity . . . '

The role of inhibition in the development of more selective motor patterns can be observed in babies and young children, and many of the more primitive patterns can be seen in monkeys and the higher apes. Before the hand and fingers become instruments of precision, the hand as a whole is used for grasping. The young baby grasps with flexion of all fingers and adduction of the thumb, and by holding the arm in flexion and pronation. At this stage, the third and fourth fingers are the strongest due to the flexed and pronated position of the arm. As extensor tone increases throughout the body musculature, the arm extends and the fingers open and the baby learns to reach out with an extended arm and grasp an object. At this stage, also, the child begins to use the arm for support. External rotation and supination of the arm and hand develop together with extension and, with the ability to supinate, the radial fingers become more active until, at about 10 months of age, the thumb and first finger become emancipated (Gesell and Amatruda, 1949). At this stage, opposition of the thumb and index finger is possible and the child can pick up small objects with them.

Inhibition of those parts of a movement which are unnecessary and might interfere with a specific activity produces the great variety of motor responses which enable the normal person to perform manual skills. The hemiplegic patient not only lacks the necessary variety of motor patterns, but is also unable to combine various patterns. For instance, he will be able either to hold or to manipulate an object which is lying on a table, but he will not be able to hold and manipulate it at the same time, or when the arm is lifted up.

Flexion and pronation of the arm make extension of wrist and fingers and abduction of fingers and thumb difficult or impossible. Recovery of movements of the fingers usually begins with the fourth and fifth finger, as in a young baby, but may not progress towards the radial side of the hand due to excessive pronation and ulnar deviation of the hand. If supination can be achieved, the patient may learn to use the thumb and all fingers. He may learn to extend and abduct his fingers and thumb when his arm is fully extended, but not when it is flexed. He may learn to supinate his forearm in flexion but, in this position, he will have difficulty in holding an object, as the total pattern of supination produces extension and abduction of the fingers. However, he may, in this position, be able to release objects while, with his arm in pronation, he may be able to grasp but not release. Opposition of the thumb and index finger is rarely achieved. Some patients may learn to grasp and release by using the whole hand, but individual and discrete movements of the fingers for manipulation of small objects need a degree of control and inhibition which is beyond the ability of most patients. In these cases, the treatment should aim mainly at making the patient use his affected hand for support, grasp and release.

The main problem in performing skilled movements is their complexity. They need constantly changing combinations of easier, and less selective movements, which are part of the more complex combinations which constitute a skill. If some, or most, of the easier movements are impossible for the patient, their more complex combinations will also be impossible. In childhood, these develop before a child is ready to use them for skilled activities. For instance, at about 9 or 10 months of age, a child can wipe, scratch, rake, poke with the index finger, pick up small objects with index finger and thumb, pull, push, wave, pat, pluck, throw and release objects. He can transfer objects from hand to hand and rub one hand with the other—just as in washing hands. He explores his mouth, face and body, and he 'fingers' objects before he can manipulate them. These are but a few examples of many easier movements all of which are necessary for later use in different combinations and with more volition for tasks such as dressing, undressing, washing, feeding and, later still, writing and drawing. These easier movements should be practised by the adult patient during the occupational therapy sessions in preparation for functional use. It would, in fact, be valuable if the occupational therapist were to analyze skills so that she might know what they entail and what is needed for their performance. She would then be able to find out which movements may be missing and arrange for the patient to practise these first.

A special field for the occupational therapist is the testing of proprioceptive, tactile and spatial sensation. In hemiplegia many motor problems are associated with sensory deficit. Therefore, improvement of discrimination of sensory modalities, such as heat, cold, shapes and textures, and different weights of objects, is of great importance. Perceptual and visio-motor training and the appreciation of 'right' and 'left' are also important aspects of her work. Testing and treatment should not be separate procedures, but should be combined, i.e. the test material used by the occupational therapist should also be used in treatment and the patient should be retested from time to time.

As physiotherapists and occupational therapists should work for the same objectives, i.e. to prepare for specific functional skills in similar ways, the techniques used in the two departments are not presented separately. Here, however, are a few illustrations to serve as examples.

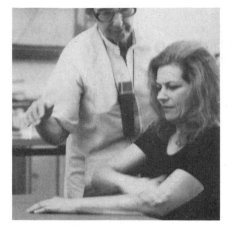

Fig. 6.54a   *The affected arm rests on the table, well forward, hand open, fingers extended. Patient should control associated reactions while rubbing the affected arm hard with sound hand. Inhibitory control of flexor spasticity by the patient.*

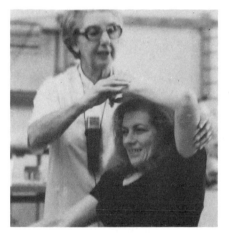

Fig. 6.54b   *The affected arm is lifted and placed palm down on the head. Alternating isolated flexion, and extension, movements of the elbow are practised. The hand should rest only lightly on the head and pressure downwards should be avoided. The elbow must neither pull forward nor down. The patient should stroke her hair lightly as in combing or smoothing it down.*

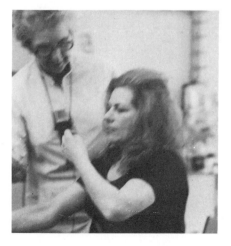

Fig. 6.54c   *Moving arm forward and up while flexing elbow supinated to bring hand to mouth. This is first practised without holding an object. Later it may be done with a utensil such as a spoon.*

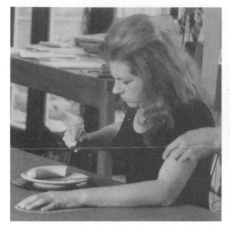

Fig. 6.55a Controlling associated reactions using right hand (the normal one) while leaving affected one flat on table, well forward, open hand (autoinhibition).
Note: Position of hand on table is marked.

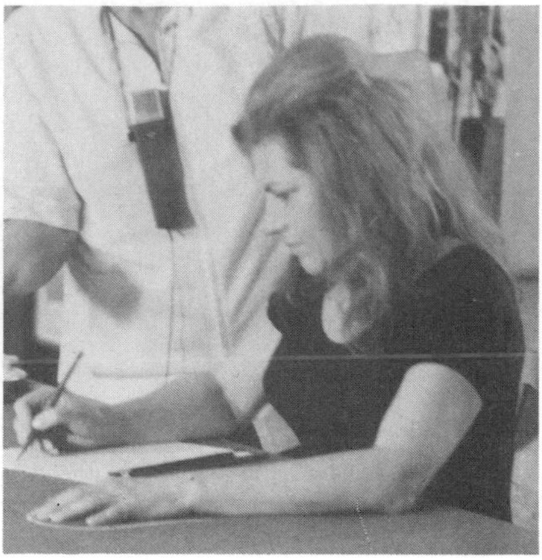

Fig. 6.55b The same activity when writing.

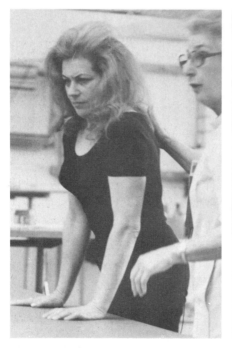

Fig. 6.56a Weightbearing on extended arms, shoulder well forward.

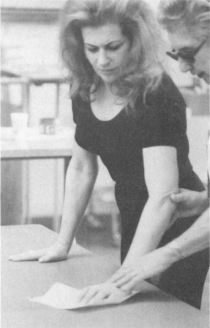

Fig. 6.56b Dusting table top with affected arm. Adduction of the arm is easier than abduction.

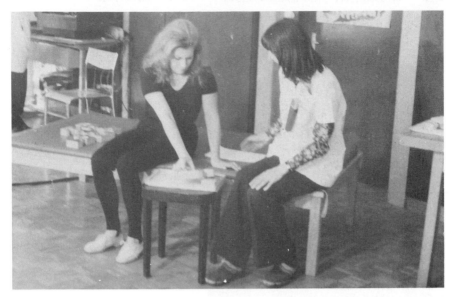

Fig. 6.57a   *Patient sits on table picking up objects with sound hand and transferring them across to the affected side. This should give the necessary rotation.*
Note: *Rotation of the shouldergirdle.*

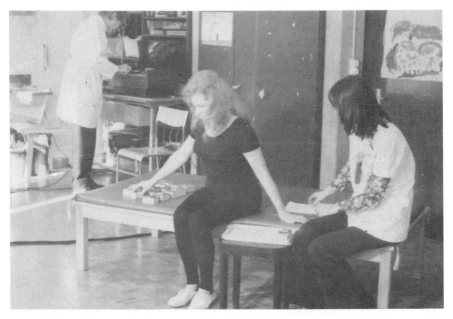

Fig. 6.57b   *While transferring objects towards the affected side, the patient supports herself on the hemiplegic arm. Associated reactions are inhibited through arm support on the affected side.*

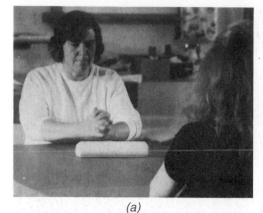

(a)

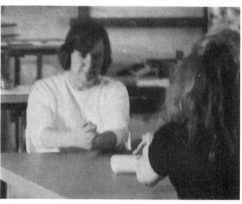

(b)

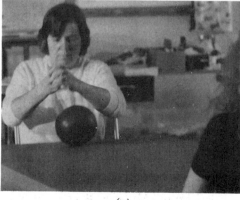

(c)

Figs. 6.58   These figures show bilateral activities.
Note: These exercises allow for group games. (a) Pushing a roll with clasped hands towards—(b) Hemiplegic patient opposite. (c) The same exercise with a ball. Now patients have to lift the arm to catch the ball before pushing it back to partner opposite.

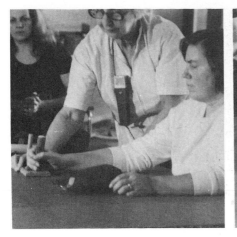

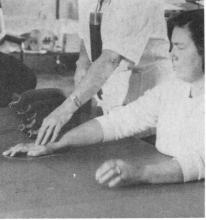

Fig. 6.59a Grasping and holding an upright stick fixed to table with the affected hand, elbow straight and shoulder well forward. This is a very useful way to avoid associated reactions while writing, eating or drawing with sound hand.

Fig. 6.59b Affected arm extended forward and maintained within chalk marks using sound hand.

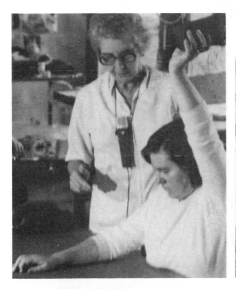

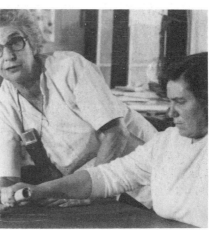

Fig. 6.59c Patient must also keep affected hand within chalk marks while raising a heavy object, such as a sand bag, with the sound arm. The weight can be increased gradually.

Fig. 6.59d Patient holding a cardboard roll with extended arm while lifting weights with sound arm.

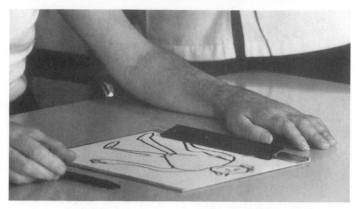

Fig. 6.60 *Drawing with sound hand and affected arm on table, shoulder well forward and hand open, fingers extended flat on table.*
Note: *Figs. 6.59a–d and 6.60 show inhibitory control exercised by the patient—autoinhibition.*

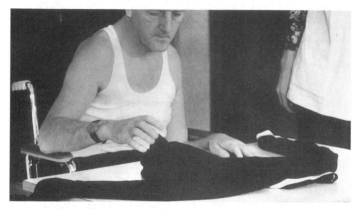

Fig. 6.61 *Preparing pullover prior to dressing to train perception. This is frequently necessary especially in left-sided hemiplegia.*

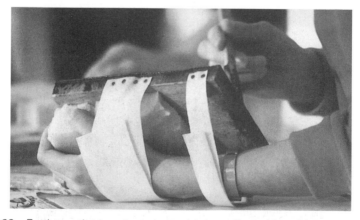

Fig. 6.62 *Putting paint to a board attached to affected hand in preparation for printing.*
Note: *The patient needs supination of the forearm for this purpose.*

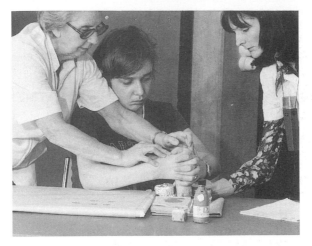

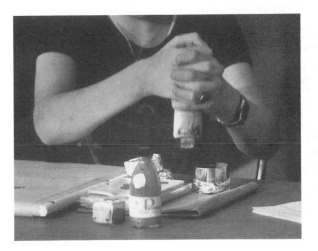

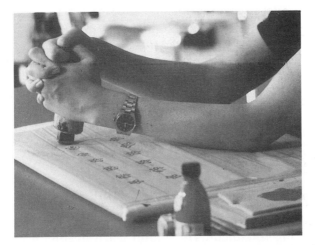

Figs. 6.63a, b, c   Printing with clasped hands showing bilateral activities.

SUMMARY OF MAIN POINTS OF TREATMENT

Assessment

This is essential at the beginning of treatment. It continues, however, during treatment and is, in fact, part of every treatment.

Reduction of spasticity by counteracting the patterns of spasticity

This results in easier and more effortless movements, without associated reactions. When the resistance of spastic antagonists has been reduced, apparently weak muscles can then contract sufficiently.

Increase of tonus

Activation of the patient by sensory stimulation, both proprioceptive and tactile, may be necessary when there is flaccidity or real weakness of muscles.

Inhibition and dissociation of total patterns

The mass patterns whether normal or abnormal, are broken up in order to obtain more selective and functional motor patterns.

Associated reactions to be avoided or inhibited

In spastic conditions patients should not be made to use effort. Arm and leg should not be treated separately, but the interaction of arm and leg through movement of the trunk must be considered.

Facilitation and stimulation

Facilitation to get balance and righting reactions, protective extension and support on the affected arm and hand, and mobile weightbearing on the leg, should be obtained.

Patient's awareness

The patient should be made aware of what he is doing, good or bad, at all times during treatment. He should learn to inhibit his spasticity (autoinhibition).

Application of techniques

1. *In spastic conditions*. Inhibition and facilitation should be done simultaneously or alternately. Voluntary activity of patient should be enlisted only when spasticity is under control. Remember that spasticity of neck and trunk influences that of the limbs (importance of rotation of trunk).
2. *In flaccid conditions*. Special techniques of stimulation may have to be given to increase tone. Voluntary activity of the patient is encouraged, but inhibition should be used if spasticity intervenes before it becomes strong.
3. *For all patients*. Importance of sensory motor re-education must be borne in mind. The patient must be made aware of the new, more normal, sensory experiences so that he learns to control his movements actively. Remember that to begin with he does not know what he is doing, i.e. when his spasticity makes him push or pull. Inhibitory control has to be handed over to the patient in easy stages by gradually and systematically reducing the control exercised by the therapist.

Feed-back between therapist and patient

The therapist should aim to get the most normal response from the patient to her handling. It is not only important that the right techniques be used, but even more so, *how* they are used. Treatment should be done slowly so that the patient can adjust himself and have time to react to what is done. The therapist must wait for his response and allow time to check up on the quality of response with regard to changes of tone and movement patterns. She should relate what she feels and observes. She should adapt her handling and choice of techniques to the patient's reactions during treatment. In this way the patient guides the therapist. It is important that more normal activity should be made possible for the patient during treatment for two reasons:

1. The patient must be, and remain, interested while being treated and enjoy success, however small.
2. Unless she produces a change for the better within a treatment session, the therapist will not know whether her treatment has been of any value or just useless. The constant evaluation of a patient's responses will show whether a certain procedure should be continued, changed or discontinued.

For the patient, treatment means learning again how to move. Learning needs repetition. Therefore, in any one treatment session, use must be made of a combination of those movement patterns which reinforce and prepare for specific functional activities. Totally unrelated movement patterns must be avoided.

CONCLUSION

The suggestions for the treatment of the hemiplegic patient given above are intended as an outline only. The handling of a patient cannot be described in greater detail, because the physiotherapist will have to develop her own technique and continuously adjust her handling of the patient to his reactions. She has to wait for his response to being placed in a position and to being moved, and her next step in treatment depends on what she feels and observes. By inhibiting abnormal reactions and facilitating more normal ones whenever possible, the patient will gradually develop more normal motor responses to her handling.

These normal active responses to being moved in different functional patterns are the same movements that he needs, and must learn to use unaided.

7

EXAMPLE OF TREATMENT—
CASE HISTORY OF A. B.

The follow-up of a patient with a residual right-sided hemiplegia who was treated daily at the Bobath Centre for a period of four months is described.

Although the techniques described here have been adapted to the needs of one particular patient they are, nevertheless, relevant to treatment in general. It is hoped that the detailed illustrations, which show very clearly the special techniques of handling and the grips used in treatment, will be of help to the practising physiotherapist. In all cases, as in the one described, constant re-evaluation of the motor handicap at various stages should be made, and the treatment adapted to the patient's progress.

CASE HISTORY

Patient A. B., aged fifty-two, suffered a cerebral vascular accident (cerebral thrombosis) three months previous to being seen for the first time. After a short period of coma, he was left with a right-sided hemiparesis and aphasia. Recovery took place slowly during the following six weeks and he regained fairly normal use of the right leg. Speech returned partially, but the right arm and hand remained paralyzed except for some feeble movements of the shoulder. From the beginning, there was no sensory impairment of hand and arm, especially no disturbance of stereognosis.

Status When First Seen

A patient of good intelligence, he was tense and depressed, very worried about the state of his arm and the inability to communicate adequately. He carried his arm in a sling, because of constant pain in the shoulder which was said to result from a capsulitis of the shoulder joint.

Head and trunk

Spasticity of the right side of the patient's neck was present with lateral flexion of the head toward the affected side. His face was turned to the left, neck and trunk were rigidly extended, and the trunk showed some side flexion to the right.

Arm

The arm appeared flaccid and hung immobile at the side of the body, adducted and internally rotated. On attempting to lift the arm, the shouldergirdle was raised with the arm in the typical total pattern of abduction and inward rotation of the arm with retraction of the shoulder, flexion of elbow and wrist with pronation of the forearm. The wrist and fingers were held in some flexion with adduction of the thumb, while the metacarpophalangeal joints were extended. There was considerable lack of range of motion and fixation of the shouldergirdle. The patient also had severe pain on passive elevation and abduction of the arm. This was probably caused by the pressure of the humeral head against the acromion, resulting from the fixation of the scapula, the lower angle not rotating properly outward and upward. This fixation of the scapula is the result of the spastic resistance of muscles connecting it with the neck, the dorsal spine and the humerus.

Leg

The leg was only slightly spastic, and the patient walked reasonably well, but the trunk was held rather immobile with lack of rotation. The patient was unable to bend the right knee when walking. At rest, the leg showed no spasticity, except for the plantar flexor muscles of the toes. When making an effort, as sitting up from supine or rolling over to prone, and particularly when walking, there was a moderate increase of spasticity throughout the leg, resulting in a temporary increased tonus as a result of associated reactions.

FIRST STAGE OF TREATMENT

Generally speaking, the ultimate aim of treatment was to guide the patient toward the development and use of latent potentialities of the affected side. This is attained by developing maximal normal functional patterns after achieving a more normal postural tone.

The first steps are to:

1. reduce flexor spasticity of the neck and trunk of the right side;
2. obtain elevation of the arm without pain by mobilizing the

shouldergirdle and counteracting the retraction, depression, and fixation of the scapula;

3.   enable the patient to hold his arm at the shoulder in many and varied positions with elbow extended.

Treatment was started with inhibition of the hyperactive depressors of the shoulder and lateral flexors of the neck. This prepared for the mobilization of the shouldergirdle and rotation of the scapula, and was done in a side-lying, sitting or standing position and was followed by full passive elevation of the arm in extension and supination (Fig. 7.1). As a result, pain gradually diminished and almost disappeared toward the end of the first month. The inhibition of the depressor muscles of the shoulder and lateral flexors of the trunk was designed to prepare the patient for independent movements of the shouldergirdle, such as shoulder shrugging in sitting and standing (Fig. 7.2).

To enable the patient to hold his arm against gravity (first with elbow extended), a technique of 'placing' was used. The patient was encouraged to hold his arm at any point throughout the full range of movement from full elevation downward; this was done in supine, sitting and standing (Fig. 7.3).

In addition, the patient had to learn to keep his elbow extended when supporting himself on his arm (Fig. 7.4); to push himself up to a sitting position, extending the elbow, and to maintain this extension when pushed by the physiotherapist (Figs. 7.5, 7.6).

Reassessment After One Month

The patient's condition and progress was reassessed after one month. In the supine position, he was now able to hold his extended arm when placed in various stages of elevation. He was free of pain on passive elevation of the arm. In sitting, he managed to support himself on an extended arm. 'Protective extension of the arm' (stretching the arm out to protect himself from falling) was now fairly well developed, but extension of the wrist was still insufficient to achieve placing of the palm of the hand on the support.

SECOND STAGE OF TREATMENT

Functional activity is not possible unless the patient can hold his arm at the shoulder in any position while moving the elbow and hand independently. Treatment, therefore, was designed to include more selective movements of the arm by a further breaking up of the spastic patterns, such as combining abduction of the arm with extension of the elbow (Fig.7.7), flexion with adduction of the arm (Fig. 7.8), and combining flexion with supination of the raised arm (Fig. 7.9).

Supination of the forearm was first practised with external rotation of the arm (Fig. 7.10). Later, supination was practised in combination with various other patterns necessary for future functional activity (Fig. 7.11).

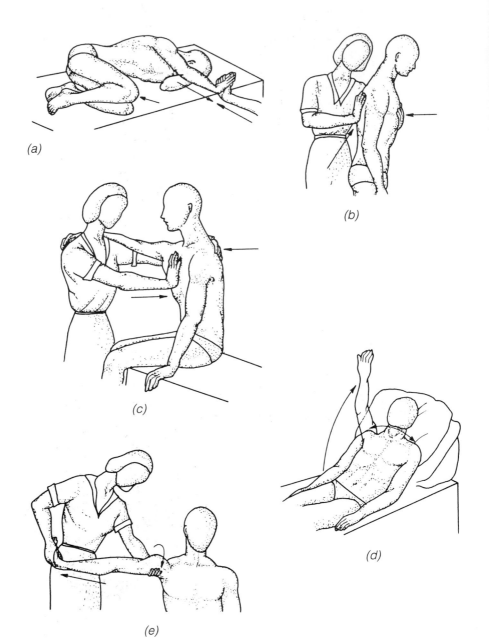

(a)

(b)

(c)

(d)

(e)

Fig. 7.1   (a) Mobilizing the shouldergirdle with extended arm. (b) Mobilizing the dorsal spine.

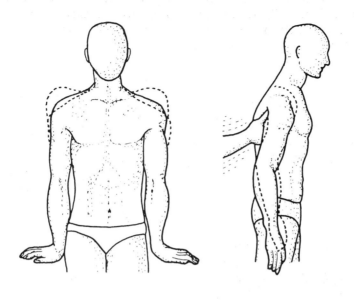

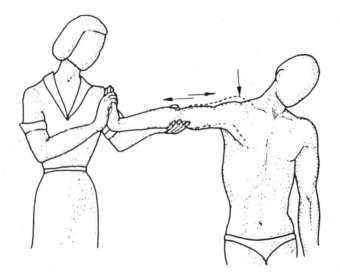

Fig. 7.2 Inhibition of the hyperactive shoulder flexors and depressors prepared the patient to attempt independent movements of the shouldergirdle such as shrugging.

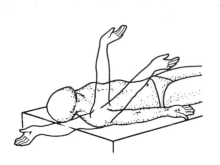

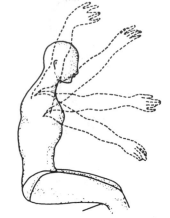

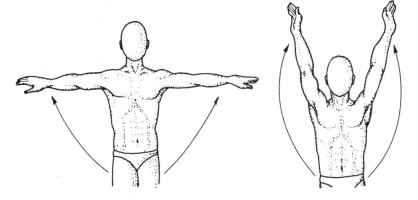

Fig. 7.3 'Placing' was used to teach the patient to hold his arm against gravity. In the three positions illustrated he was asked to hold his arm at various points throughout the range of downward motion.

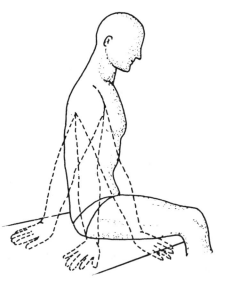

Fig. 7.4 Supporting the body in the sitting position with the extended elbow and the hand in different positions is a prerequisite to more advanced balancing exercises.

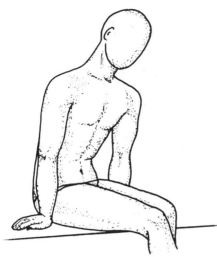

Fig. 7.5 Sitting 'push-ups' to full elbow extension are an early exercise.

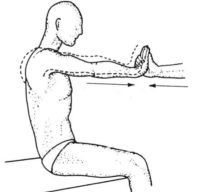

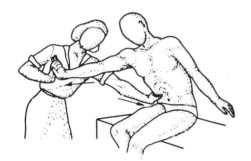

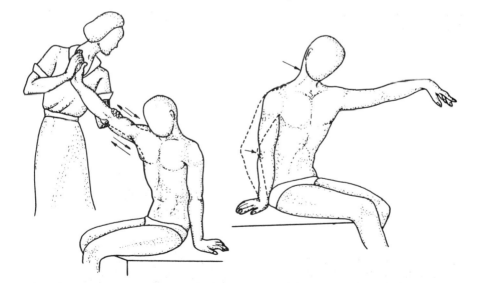

Fig. 7.6   The patient learned to keep his elbow extended against the 'pull-push' of the therapist.

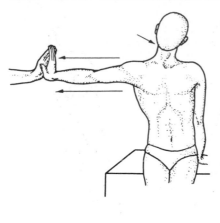

Fig. 7.7 Abduction of the arm and extension of the elbow breaks up the typical spastic pattern.

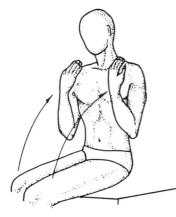

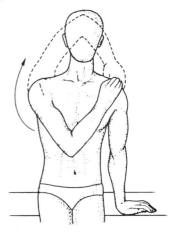

Fig. 7.8 Flexion and adduction combinations further break up the patterns of spasticity.

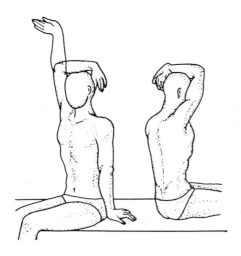

Fig. 7.9 Selective movements of the arm such as a combination of flexion with supination, with the arm elevated, were used to break up the total spastic pattern.

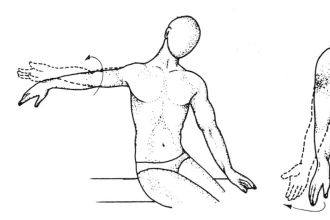

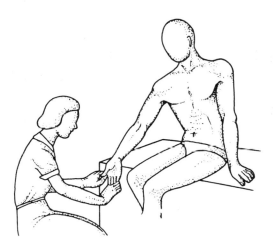

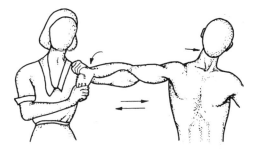

Fig. 7.10   Inhibition of flexor spasticity and supination of the forearm with the shoulder in external rotation is a pattern which is basic to obtaining future functional activity.

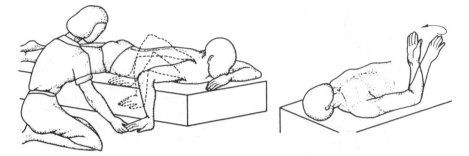

Fig. 7.11 Supination of the forearm must also be used with other shoulder motions, as depicted, to prepare the patient for functional activity. Supination of the forearm is practised with or without weightbearing.

Second Assessment

Reassessment after a further month of treatment revealed that the patient was now able to perform a number of functional movements in normal patterns. He could shake hands requiring flexion and extension of the elbow without abduction at the shoulder (Fig.7.12). He could put his hand on the table (requiring first flexion, then extension of the elbow while pushing the extended arm forward). He had, however, to be told exactly how to perform each movement at every stage or he would automatically return to the former pattern of abduction, flexion and pronation. Frequent repetition was necessary to imprint the new pattern on his mind. The first movements he could perform occurred spontaneously, i.e. automatically rather than voluntarily and were motions of expression such as: 'I don't care!' (shoulder shrugging with flexion and supination of the arm); 'Oh my God!' (hand on forehead); 'Whatever next!' (clasping hands together). These movements were done more successfully when his left hand was initially restrained and prevented from moving.

Although the patient was able to raise his arm above his head laterally and upward (not yet forward and up), it was still difficult to lift his arm with a flexed elbow and supinated wrist, as when moving his hand to the opposite shoulder or when lifting his hand to touch the crown of his head (Fig. 7.13).

He could supinate the forearm in all positions, i.e. supine, sitting and standing, but only with a total pattern of outward rotation of the arm, retraction at the shoulder, and side flexion of the trunk. He pronated with inward rotation of the arm, protraction of the shoulder, and raising of the shouldergirdle. In spite of the improvement of voluntary function during and immediately following treatment, the patient still held his arm motionless at his side throughout the day. In fact, he seemed to 'forget' the arm.

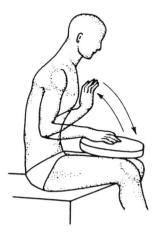

Fig. 7.12 *After two months of treatment the patient could perform some functional movements requiring selective extension and flexion of the elbow without abduction at the shoulder, e.g. shaking hands or beating a drum.*

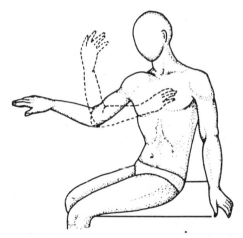

Fig. 7.13 *The motion shown here, involving supination of the forearm, flexion of the elbow and forward flexion or adduction of the shoulder, was difficult to achieve.*

THIRD STAGE OF TREATMENT

The aim of treatment at this stage was, therefore, to make the patient aware of the arm as part of his whole body, and to make him use the arm. He was not only made to move the arm against his trunk, but also to use the arm as a point of fixation for movements of the trunk against his arm. The following activities were practised: getting up from, and sitting down on a chair, or from a bed, moving from upright kneeling to four-foot kneeling, and into standing, crawling, weight-bearing, balancing and lunging (Fig. 7.14).

Repeated rotation of the patient's spine and shouldergirdle was practised to inhibit flexor spasticity of the shouldergirdle and arm to facilitate the free swing of this arm. (Fig. 7.15).

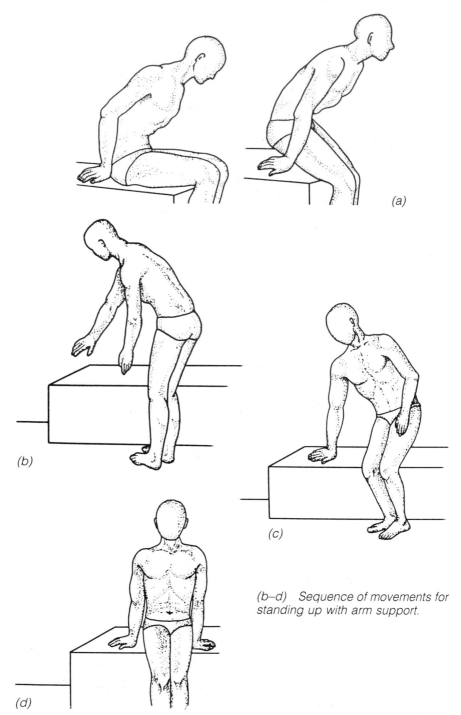

(a)

(b)

(c)

(b–d) *Sequence of movements for standing up with arm support.*

(d)

Fig. 7.14   *Activities designed to make the patient aware of his arm as part of his whole body are depicted here and on the following pages. (a) arm support with extension for pushing up to take weight on legs.*

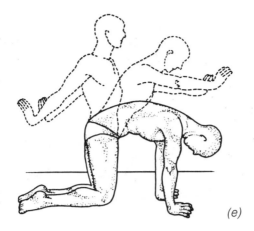

(e)

(e)   Sequence of movements for standing up from kneeling.

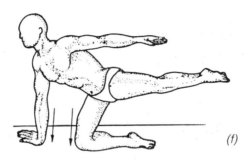

(f)

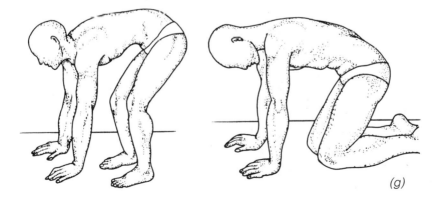

(g)

(f–k)   Weightbearing on affected arm and leg.

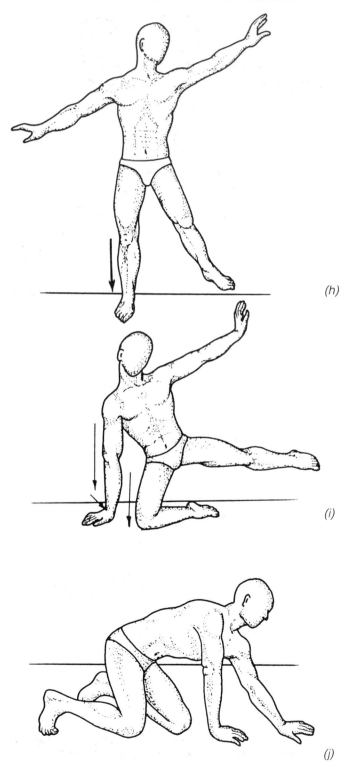

(h)

(i)

(j)

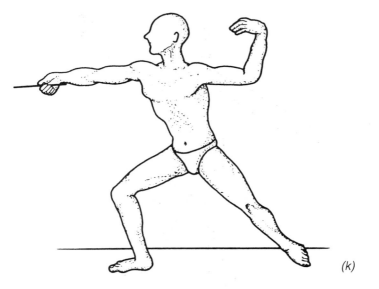

(k)

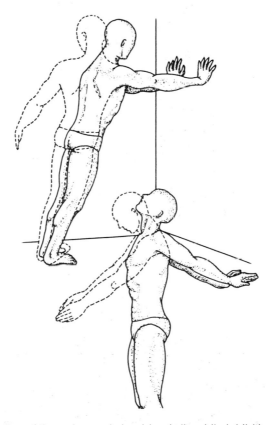

Fig. 7.15   Rotation of the spine and shouldergirdle while inhibiting the resistance of the spastic shoulder muscle aids free swinging of the arms.

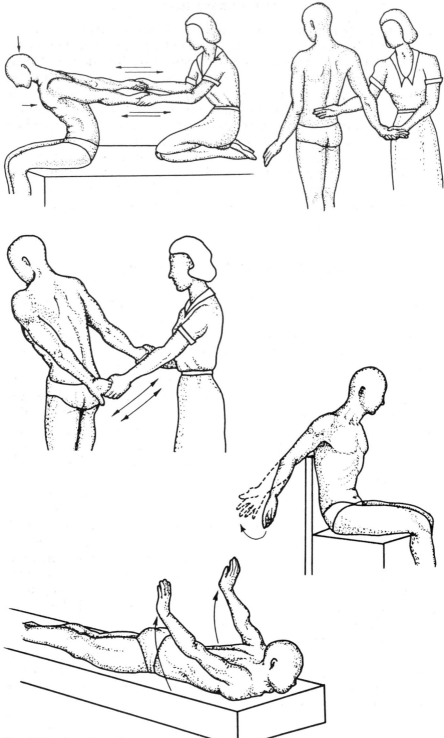

Fig. 7.15 (continued)

Third Assessment

On reassessing the patient after another month of treatment, there was further improvement. The patient had better active motion of his arm and hand and he held his arm normally during the day. When moved passively, the arm felt lighter and the shoulder was less retracted. The patient could lift his arm to touch the head or face, but he had to do this rather quickly as he was, as yet, unable to control every stage of the movement. He could extend and flex his wrist when lying supine, arm at his side, elbow flexed to 90°, forearm vertical.

There were slight active movements of the fingers, mainly of the thumb and fifth finger, but they could as yet only be obtained with the arm extended, supported, and held raised at the shoulder. All movements of wrist and fingers were still easier when done in supine than in any other position.

FOURTH STAGE OF TREATMENT

While the treatment as described above was continued, emphasis was put on obtaining selective movements of the wrist and fingers with extension and abduction of fingers and thumb, at the same time inhibiting the pattern of pronation, flexion of elbow and wrist, and adduction of fingers and thumb. This inhibition had been carried out previously in all positions using the grips shown in Figs 7.18 and 7.10. Extension of the wrist was first practised with an extended elbow, the arm held by the physiotherapist, and later with a flexed elbow (Fig. 7.16). Extension of the wrist and fingers with flexion of the metacarpal joints and abduction of the thumb was practised, using weight and pressure on the hand, followed by the same movement done actively (Fig. 7.17).

When treatment at the Centre was discontinued, the patient could grasp and release an object. He could move his extended index finger and could abduct, flex and extend his thumb. The third and fourth fingers were still inactive, although they showed weak movements directly after treatment. The patient left at the end of four months' treatment. A report on the patient's progress six months later revealed spasticity as minimal. The patient could move his wrist at almost normal speed and finger motion improved daily. He could abduct and adduct his extended fingers and oppose his thumb to all fingers, but all fingers would flex when opposing the thumb.

A month later, correspondence revealed that the patient was 'doing new movement with his fingers' each day. He could move the fingers separately, and he had begun to use his hand spontaneously to help himself in everyday activities.

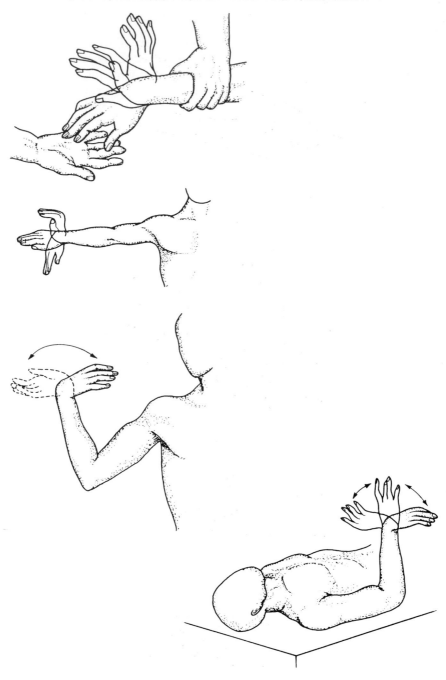

Fig. 7.16 During the fourth stage of treatment, emphasis shifted towards obtaining active movements of the wrist and fingers. The pattern of pronation and flexion of the elbow and wrist and adduction of the fingers had to be inhibited. Extension of the wrist was carried out first with the extended elbow and later with a flexed elbow.

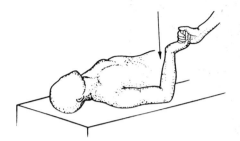

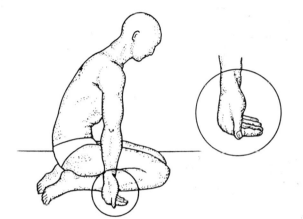

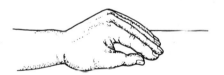

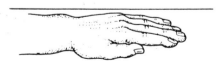

Fig. 7.17 Extension of the wrist and fingers with flexion at the metacarpo-
phalangeal joints was performed with assistance, and then actively by the patient.

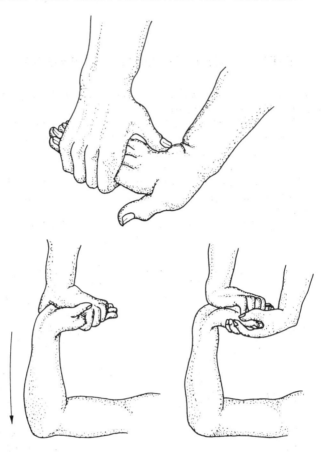

Fig. 7.18   Grips used to carry out exercises which inhibit unwanted activity.
See also: *the final drawing in Fig. 7.10, p. 169.*

CONCLUSION

This patient was chosen as an example despite the fact that he was still in the period of spontaneous recovery, because his case presented the possibility of describing and illustrating a great variety of techniques used in treatment.

The patient's arm and hand had shown no sign of spontaneous recovery until treatment was started three months after the cerebral vascular accident. The arm and hand responded surprisingly well once physiotherapy was begun. Results obtained in this case by intensive treatment should encourage physiotherapists to persevere, especially with patients having little or no sensory deficit.

It must be emphasized that the treatment has proved of great value in improving the condition of patients with residual hemiplegia of many years' standing.

REFERENCES AND FURTHER READING

Banks M. A. (1986). *International Perspectives in Physiotherapy*, pp. 99–128. Edinburgh: Churchill Livingstone.

Basmajian J. V. (1962). *Muscles Alive: Their Function Revealed by Electromyography*, pp. 103–5, 158, 159. London: Ballière, Tindall & Cox.

Basmajian, J. V. (1969). Recent advances in the functional anatomy of the upper limb. *Am. J. Phys. Med.*, **48**, No. 4.

Basmajian J. V., Kukulka C. G., Narayan M. G. *et al.* (1975). Biofeedback treatment of the foot drop after stroke. *Arch. Phys. Med. Rehab.*, **56**, (June), pp. 231–6.

Beevor C. E. (1904). *The Croonian Lectures*. London: Adlard & Son.

Bernstein N. (1967). *The Co-ordination and Regulation of Movements*, pp. 111–13. Oxford: Pergamon Press.

Bobath B. (1969). The treatment of neuromuscular disorders by improving patterns of co-ordination. *Physiotherapy*, **55**, 1, 18–22.

Bobath B. (1985). *Abnormal Postural Reflex Activity Caused by Brain Lesions*, 3rd edn. London: William Heinemann Medical Books.

Bobath K. (1959). The effect of treatment by reflex inhibition and facilitation in cerebral palsy. *Folia Psychiatrica, Neurologica et Neurochirugica Neerlandica*, **62**, 448.

Bobath K. (1966). *Motor Deficit in Patients with Cerebral Palsy*. Clinics in Developmental Medicine, No. 23, p. 24. London: Spastic International Medical Publications in association with William Heinemann Medical Books.

Bobath K. (1971). The problem of spasticity in the treatment of patients with lesions of the upper motor neurone. In *Proceedings for the 6th International Congress of the World Confederation for Physical Therapy*, Amsterdam, April/May 1970. (Prakke H. J., Prakke H. M. G., eds.) pp. 459–64. Assen: Van Gorcum.

Bobath K. (1980). *A Neurophysiological Basis for the Treatment of Cerebral Palsy*, 2nd edn. Clinics in Developmental Medicine, No. 75. London: Spastics International Medical Publications in association with William Heinemann Medical Books.

Brain W. R. (1927). On the significance of the flexor posture of the upper limb in hemiplegia, with an account of the quadrupedal extensor reflex. *Brain*, **50**, 113–37.

Brain W. R. (1956). *Diseases of the Nervous System*, p. 40. Oxford: Oxford University Press.

Brunnstrom S. (1956a). Methods used to elicit, reinforce and co-ordinate muscular response in adult patients with hemiplegia. In *APTA OVR Institute Papers*.

Brunnstrom S. (1956b). Associated reactions of the upper extremity in adult patients with hemiplegia. *Phys. Ther. Rev.*, **35**, 4.

Brunnstrom S. (1970). *Movement Therapy in Hemiplegia: a Neurophysiological Approach*. New York: Harper and Row.

Carr J. H., Shepherd R. B. (1987). *A Motor Relearning Programme for Stroke*, 2nd edn. London: William Heinemann Medical Books.

Clemessen S. (1951). Some studies on muscle tone. *Proc. Roy. Soc. Med.*, **44**, 637.

Coghill G. E. (1936). Correlated anatomical and phsyiological studies of the growth of the nervous system of Amphybias. *J. Comp. Neur.*, Pts. I–XII.

Coghill G. E. Quoted in 'Cats' Economy of Effort'. The World of Science. *Illustrated London News*, Feb. 27 (1954).

Critchley M. (1954). Discussion of volitional movement. *Roy. Soc. Med.*, **47**, 593–4.

Davies P. M. (1985). Shoulder problems associated with hemiplegia. In *Steps to Follow*, pp. 206–341. Berlin: Springer Verlag.

Davis S. (1977). Shoulder-hand syndrome in a hemiplegic population: a five-year retrospective study. *Arch. Phys. Med. Rehab.*, **58**, 353–6.

Dimitrijevic M. R., Fagnal J., Sherwood A. M., *et al.* (1981). Activation on paralysed leg flexors and extensors in patients during gait after stroke. *Scand. J. Rehab. Med.*, **13**, 109–15.

Drachman D. A. (1967). Disorders of tone. *Am. J. Phys. Med.*, **46**, 1.

Eccles J. C. (1973). *The Understanding of the Brain.* New York: McGraw-Hill Book Co.

Eggars O. (1983). *Occupational Therapy in the Treatment of Adult Hemiplegia.* London: William Heinemann Medical Books.

Fog E., Fog M. (1963). *Cerebral Inhibition Examined by Associated Movements.* Little Club Clinics in Developmental Medicine, No. 10, p. 52. London: National Spastics Society Medical Education and Information Unit in association with William Heinemann Medical Books.

Gardiner D. (1963). *The Principles of Exercise Therapy*, p. 78. London: G. Bell & Sons.

Gautier-Smith P. C. (1976). Clinical management of spastic state. *Physiotherapy*, **62**, 326–8.

Gesell A., Amatruda C. S. (1949). *Developmental Diagnosis.* New York: Paul B. Hoeber.

Gatev V. (1972). The role of inhibition in the development of motor co-ordination in early childhood. *Dev. Med. Child Neurol.*, **14**, 336–41.

Gee, Z. L., Passarella P. M. (1985). *Nursing Care of the Stroke Patient. A Therapeutic Approach.* Pittsburgh: American Rehabilitation Education Network, (AREN Publications).

Goff B. (1969). The application of recent advances in neurophysiology to Miss M. Rood's concept of neuromuscular facilitation. *Physiotherapy* **55**, (January), 409–19.

Grasty P. (1985). *Home Care for the Stroke Patient in the Early Days.* London: The Chest, Heart and Stroke Association.

Hawker S., Squires A. (1980). *Return to Mobility*, 2nd edn. London: The Chest, Heart and Stroke Association.

Horak P. E. (1987). Clinical measurement of postural control in adults. *Am. Phys. Ther.*, **67**, 12, 1881–5.

Housmanova Petrusewicz (1959). Interaction in simultaneous motor function. *A.M.D. Arch. Neurol. Psych.*, **81**, 173–81.

Isaacs B. (1977). Stroke research and the phsyiotherapist. *Physiotherapy*, **63**, 11, 366–7.

Jensen G. M. (1989). Qualitative methods in physical therapy research. A form of disciplined inquiry. *Phys. Ther.*, **69**, 6, 492–500.

Johnstone M. (1980). *Home Care for the Stroke Patient.* Edinburgh: Churchill Livingstone.

Kabat H. (1953). Proprioceptive facilitation techniques for treatment of paralysis. *Phys. Ther. Rev.,* **33**, 2.

Kelly, R. E., Gautier-Smith P. C. (1959). Intrathecal phenol in the treatment of reflex spasms and spasticity. *Lancet,* **ii**, 1102–5.

Knott M. (1967). Introduction to and philosophy of neuromuscular facilitation. *Physiotherapy,* **53**, 1, 2.

Knott M., Voss D. E. (1973). *Proprioceptive Neuromuscular Facilitation.* New York: Harper & Row, Hoeber Medical Division.

Lane R. E. J. (1978). Facilitation of weight transferences in the stroke patient. *Physiotherapy,* **64**, 9, 260–4.

Magnus R. (1924). *Koerperstellung* p. 45: Berlin: Julius Springer.

Magnus R. (1926). Some results of studies in the physiology of posture. *Lancet,* **ii**, 531–6, 585–8.

Magoun H. W., Rhines H. (1946). Inhibitory mechanism in bulbar reticular formation. *J. Neurophys.,* **9**, 165–71.

Magoun H. W., Rhines H. (1948). *Spasticity, the Stretch Reflex and the Extra-pyramidial Systems.* Springfield, Illinois: C. C. Thomas.

Nathan P. W. (1980). Factors affecting spasticity. *Int. Rehab. J.,* **2**, 1, 1–40.

Rademaker G. G. (1935). *Reactions Labyrinthiques et Equilibré.* Paris: Masson et Cie.

Reinhold M. (1951). Some clinical aspects of human cortical function. *Brain,* **74**, 4.

Reynolds Glenn C., Brunnstrom S. (1959). Problems of sensory motor learning in evaluation and treatment of adult hemiplegia patients. *Rehab. Lit.,* **20**, 6.

Rood M. S. (1956). *Am. J. Occ. Ther.,* **10**, 4.

Riddoch C., Buzzard E. F. (1921). Reflex movements and postural reactions in quadriplegia and hemiplegia, with special reference to those of the upper limb. *Brain,* **44**, 397.

Rushworth G. (1980). Some pathophysiological aspects of spasticity. *Int. J. Rehab. Med.,* **13**, 109–15.

Schaltenbrand G. (1927). The development of human motility and motor disturbances. *Bull. N.Y. Acad. Med.,* **3**, 54.

Schaltenbrand G. (1928). The development of human motility and motor disturbances. *Arch. Neur. Psych.,* **20**, 720.

Semans S. (1965). Treatment of neurological disorders, concept and systems. *Am. Phys. Ther. Ass.,* **45**, 1, 11–16.

Sherrington C. S. (1913). Reflex inhibition as a factor in the co-ordination of movements and postures. *Quart. J. Exp. Physiol.,* **6**, 251.

Sherrington C. S. (1947). *The Integrative Action of the Nervous System,* pp. 67–9. Cambridge: Cambridge University Press.

Souza L. H., Langton Hewer R., Lynn P. A., *et al.* (1980) Assessment of recovery of arm control in hemiplegic stroke patients. *Int. Rehab. Med.,* **2**, 1, 1–40.

Thrush D. (1976). *Mod. Geriatr.,* **6**, 6, 11.

Triptree V. J., Harrison M. A. (1980). The use of sensor pads in the treatment of hemiplegia. *Physiotherapy,* **66,** 9.

Twitchell T. E. (1951). The restoration of motor function following hemiplegia in man. *Brain,* **74**, 4, 443.

Twitchell T. E. (1954). Sensory factors in purposive movements. *J. Neurophysiol.*, **XVIII**, 3, 249.

Twitchell T. E. (1961). The clinical differentiation and physiological nature of increased resistance to passive movement. *Cerebral Palsy Bulletin*, **3**, 1, 110–6.

Uexküell J. von (1905). Muscle tone studies II. The movements of the brittlestar. *Z. Biol.*, **46**, 1–37.

Walshe F. M. R. (1923). On certain tonic or postural reflexes in hemiplegia with special reference to the so-called associated movements. *Brain*, **46**, 1, 2–33.

Walshe F. M. R. (1948) *Critical Studies in Neurology*, p. 215. Edinburgh: Livingstone.

Walters C. E. (1967). Interaction of the body and its segments. *Am. J. Phys. Med.*, **46**, 1.

Weisz St. (1938). Studies in equilibrium reactions. *J. Nerv. Ment. Dis.*, **88**, 153, 160–2.

Williams, R., Tufts L., Minuk T. (1988). Evaluation of two support methods for the subluxed shoulder of hemiplegia patients. *J. Am. Phys. Ther. Ass.*, **68**, 209–1213.

Zador J. (1938). Les Réactions d'Equilibrés Chez l'Homme. Paris: Masson et Cie.

INDEX